Fat, Fatigued and Fed Up?

How Metabolic Syndrome Is Destroying Your Life

Dr. Trent Camp & Dr. Dane Donohue

Fat, Fatigued and Fed Up?
How Metabolic Syndrome Is Destroying Your Life
ISBN: 978-0-9913939-4-7
By Dr. Trent Camp and Dr. Dane Donohue

1st Printing, February 2014
Printed in the United States of America

Dedication

I'd like to dedicate this book to my family, friends and patients whose love and support gives me a reason to do what I love. I've found that the greatest happiness in the world comes from serving others in a way that respects one's own values and talents.

I'd like to acknowledge first my co-author, Dr. Trent Camp. Everyone in life needs a coach, a mentor, a person that sees more in you than you see in yourself. For me, that person is my accountability partner and dear friend Dr. Trent Camp.

To my twin sister and co-developer of the life-saving program, 8 Weeks to Wellness, your passion and caring has always been a North Star for me. It has guided me in the direction of serving others before myself. To my incredible family of Chiropractors and Chiropractic fans, it hasn't always been easy to be a Chiropractic family. We hold values and principles that often contradict the norms of society. We believe that having belief in one's own healing ability, accompanied by behavior that honors the body, mind and spirit, are much more powerful than any fistful of pills.

To my wife Jill, who has always stood by my side through my ups and downs, there has never been another person, nor will there be, that I respect more. Finally, to my two sons, Chris and Shane, I say to you two growing men, go find a purpose in life that serves others, helps the suffering and gives you immense pleasure and happiness and you will honor the God that put you on this earth.

Contents

1

Introduction

Metabolic Syndrome

"It is important for Americans to recognize that, despite all of the fancy gimmicks and perceived power of modern medicine, the largest explosion of preventable, chronic diseases ever in the history of mankind has occurred as a direct result of modern medicine and scientific reductionism. Modern medicine is not an antidote for the incredible harms caused by the modern food industry, but it is an effective distraction." ~ Charles C. Harpe

What Is Metabolic Syndrome?

Metabolic syndrome, also called Syndrome X, is the leading cause of death in the United States. It is a condition which left untreated will lead to chronic disease and eventually death. People are dying differently today than years ago. No longer are we dying of infectious diseases like the bubonic plague, scarlet fever or polio. People are dying of chronic diseases like:

- Heart Disease (597,689 deaths in 2011)
- Cancer (574,743 deaths in 2011)
- Obesity related diseases such as diabetes (69,071 deaths in 2011)[1]

In fact, 50% of the American population will die this year from either heart disease or cancer. Over 44% of us will die before the young age of 74. You are three to four times more likely to die of cardiovascular disease if you have metabolic syndrome even when the presence of other risk factors are taken into account.[2]

Understanding metabolic syndrome and how to prevent and cure it is the key to knowing if you are on the path to a health or on the path towards early chronic disease and death (see figure A on next page).

Discovering metabolic syndrome in a patient can be very valuable in preventing a health crisis. It is like having a road map that shows us where a patient will eventually arrive unless we take them off the road they're on, thereby providing a new (and healthier) destination.

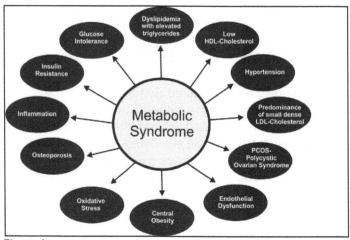

Figure A

Forty percent of the population over 40 years old have metabolic syndrome, twenty percent over the age of 20 have it and the most startling statistic is that 50% or **one in two** Americans over the age of 60 have metabolic syndrome.[3] However, most do not know anything about it and therefore do not know that they have a time bomb ticking away which *can* be defused!

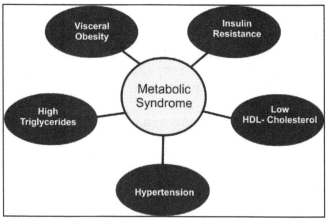

Figure B

Certain blood chemistry along with physical components can determine if a person has, or is getting, metabolic syndrome (see figure B on previous page). Once discovered, lifestyle changes can be made in order to prevent potential illness from becoming full blown. Metabolic syndrome is tricky to diagnose because the person gradually develops the disease. Most people suffering from metabolic syndrome or pre-metabolic syndrome are completely unaware of it, but if not corrected, in time will likely lead to diseases such as:

- Diabetes
- Stroke
- Heart disease
- Cancer
- And a host of other ill-health conditions

One of the key indicators and problems with metabolic syndrome is insulin resistance. Simply stated, this happens when there is a problem converting the foods you eat into the energy you need. When you eat, your body breaks down your food into glucose which then travels from the bloodstream and is supposed to go into your cells. Glucose, also called blood sugar, can either be used as energy or stored as fat. This energy is what is required for every function in the body. In order for the body to use the glucose for energy or to store it, it needs insulin. Insulin is a hormone, produced in the pancreas. When functioning properly and proper diet is maintained, the pancreas secretes the right amount of insulin needed to transfer and process the glucose created from our food. But when the body has insulin resistance, it hinders this transfer and that is where the problems begin.[4]

Most people think about diabetes when they hear the word insulin. Diabetes occurs when there is a problem with the natural production of insulin in our body.

Insulin Deficiency

In type 1 Diabetes, the body's immune system doesn't work properly. Instead of creating the insulin needed, the body attacks the cells that produce insulin, leaving the body with no way to get the glucose into the cells. This type of diabetes is non-reversible and usually identified at a very young age.[5]

Type 2 Diabetes is the most common form of diabetes. About 90-95% of people have this type of diabetes. With this type, the body doesn't make enough insulin or the cells of the body don't recognize the insulin to get all the glucose out of the bloodstream and into the cells.[6] This condition can worsen over time if changes in lifestyle are not made. Even when controlled, diabetes lessens a person's lifespan up to 6 years.[7] Diabetes is the number one cause of blindness in adults, the number one cause of kidney failure, the number one cause of amputations and the seventh leading cause of death in the United States.[8]

Insulin Resistance

When insulin is sufficient, it activates the cell to draw glucose into itself. Think of this scenario to illustrate (where "cars" are our cells, "gasoline" is our glucose and the "fuel pump" is our insulin): Our cars run on gasoline. In order to get the gasoline into our cars we need the fuel pumps. But what happens if many of the fuel pumps are broken, and just don't work? There are fewer avenues to get the gas from the gas tanks into our cars. We may have to wait a long time to get the gasoline we need, and without it, we don't have the fuel to run our car properly.

If there isn't enough insulin for the glucose requirement, the glucose remains in the bloodstream, and is unable to be used for energy. The body converts the excess glucose into triglycerides (which is why you should know your triglyceride number) and ultimately stores this excess glucose as fat which gets distributed around our body, particularly around our mid-section. We call this fat VAT, visceral adipose tissue because it is the fat that engulfs your viscera (organs).[9] Also, glucose is one of the few molecules that can cross the blood-brain barrier. So when it is left uncontrolled and there are high levels of glucose in our blood stream, it damages our nerve tissue. This is why we see so many neurological complications with diabetes. This is often referred to as diabetic neuropathy. This is what happens when you have metabolic syndrome.

The Five Factors of Metabolic Syndrome

There are five factors that are attributed with metabolic syndrome.[10] Unfortunately you only need to have three out of the five to have it, and an increased risk for many different diseases. And chances are if you have even two of them, the third is on its way. These factors are:

- Abdominal Obesity
- High Triglycerides
- Low HDL
- Elevated Blood Pressure
- Blood Glucose Level of over 100

Let's look at each of these.

Abdominal Obesity

This means that you carry your excess weight in your abdomen. It is figured by measuring the *largest* part of your waist, not where you wear your pants. You are positive for this factor if you are male and the largest measurement of your waist area is 40 inches or more, or if you're female and your largest waist measurement is 35 inches or more.

High Triglycerides

Triglycerides are blood fat.[11] They occur when you eat sugary or fatty foods. You may also have a genetic predisposition for high triglycerides. Triglycerides are measured by a blood test after a 12-hour fast. If your triglycerides are 150 or greater, you have this risk factor. When your diet is high in fats and sugars and your body doesn't burn them off or use them, the result is thicker blood. When your blood gets thick, it is harder to move through your body.[12]

Low HDL

HDL stands for high density lipoprotein and it is considered the *good* cholesterol. It's the job of HDL to scour the bloodstream and transport harmful cholesterol to the liver. When you have high HDL your risk of heart disease decreases. You qualify for this risk factor of metabolic syndrome when your HDL is less than 40 for a man or less than 50 for a woman.[13]

- *Note: if your Triglyceride to HDL ratio is greater than 3:1 this is a big risk factor for cardiovascular disease. This ratio is more accurate to determine your risk for heart disease than simply looking at your cholesterol level.*[14]

Elevated Blood Pressure

You qualify for metabolic syndrome if your blood pressure is greater than 130/85. Normal blood pressure is usually 120/80 or less, and 130/85 may not be significantly high but these numbers indicate pre-hypertension and it means you are at risk.

People know that high blood pressure is bad. However, most of the time, they don't know why. Think of it like this, if I am trying to get fluid to flow through a tube, the smaller the diameter of the tube, the higher the pressure needs to be to push fluid through that tube, correct? What pumps blood through our blood vessels (our tubes)? The correct answer is our heart and so when your blood vessels are narrowing through the process known as "arteriosclerosis" or hardening of the arteries, caused by metabolic syndrome, your heart has to strain harder to push blood through your blood vessels. This is what increases your blood pressure and why it's so important to know your baseline blood pressure. Also, arteriosclerosis causes your blood vessels to become hard and less elastic and can rupture under the increased pressure. This is what is known as a *heart attack* or *brain attack* (stroke).

Blood Glucose Level of over 100

Blood glucose or sugar is tested after a 12-hour fast to accurately determine its count. Blood sugar is considered normal if it is between 60 and 120. But when your blood sugar goes over 100, your risk for heart disease increases.[15] In fact, for each number over 100 you have an increased percentage point of getting heart disease. For instance, if your blood sugar is 101, you have a 1% increased risk for heart disease. If it's 110, you have a 10% increased risk.

These five factors described above are all somewhat similar to each other in that they all affect the blood and fat in your body and are also affected by diet and activity. When your body is unable to help you convert your blood sugar into energy, it sits in your bloodstream, expands your waist, sludges your blood and makes activities more difficult for you. Additionally, it will be heading you toward many life-threatening illnesses.

If I Have Metabolic Syndrome, Am I Doomed?

Having metabolic syndrome means you are at greater risk for heart disease, cancer and obesity-related conditions such as diabetes. But being aware that you have a health condition means you can take the necessary actions to heal the condition. The more aware you are about how your lifestyle affects your health, the quicker you can take steps to prevent these illnesses from occurring. That's why we wrote this book. *Metabolic syndrome can be reversed.* Take action to get healthier and every part of your health will change as well. You will:

- Have more energy
- Sleep more soundly
- Handle stressful situations more easily
- Have stable moods
- Be more active
- Lose unnecessary weight and/or gain muscle mass
- Have greater immunity and get sick less often
- Life a healthier life

- Have better relationships
- Be able to physically participate with your children and grandchildren
- Have more independence later in life
- Live longer
- Use less medication
- Have fewer hospital and doctor visits

According to the EPIC study done in Europe on over a half million people, there are four simple behaviors that can reduce your risk of cancer and metabolic syndrome.[16] These behaviors include:

- Not Smoking
- 3 ½ hours of exercise each week
- Having a Body Mass Index (BMI) of less than 30 (A BMI of 30 or more is considered obese)
- Eating a Healthy Diet

Let's discuss these briefly.

Not Smoking

Not smoking provides many benefits including reducing blood pressure. A person is at greater risk for many diseases when they smoke because smoking is a major cause for coronary heart disease. The more and the longer you smoke, the greater your risk. In fact, people who smoke a pack of cigarettes a day have more than twice the risk for a heart attack than a non-smoker.[17]

Exercising Three to Four Hours a Week

The Centers for Disease Control and Prevention recommend 30 minutes of exercise at least five days a week. This will increase your heart health, decrease your blood pressure and help eliminate excess calories that need to be burned off. With activity, your body functions more efficiently, weight is better managed and cholesterol is reduced. But not all exercise is equal. In order to reap the maximum benefits from a workout, you should use a heart rate monitor and make sure you are reaching the proper levels for your age and weight. The three forms of exercise that all good exercise programs include are: Weight Training, Flexibility and Mobility Training, and Cardiovascular or Aerobic Training. We'll cover this in more detail in our chapter on exercise.

Body Mass Index

Body mass index is measured from your height and weight. There are ranges that will categorize you as underweight, healthy, overweight and obese.[18] The chart itself though doesn't measure your body fat so it can be misleading, but in general it can be useful for determining if you are in a danger range, which is the obese range (BMI over 30) or morbidly obese range (BMI over 40).

Eating a Healthy Diet

Our body takes our food and breaks it down into energy. When we eat healthy foods such as lean proteins, nuts and seeds, fruits and vegetables, the food is broken down and takes a while to convert to glucose. But when our foods are high in sugar and low in fiber, there is too much sugar to process at one time and therefore our insulin is stressed and cannot get the glucose into our cells as fast as it arrives. In this case the body stores the extra glucose as fat. This is what happens with processed and refined foods and why they tax our bodies.

Overcoming Metabolic Syndrome

You *can* overcome metabolic syndrome. The three fairly simple factors it takes to do so are:

- Think Better
- Eat Better
- Move Better

Living a Life of Wellness

The 8 Weeks to Wellness® program was developed to help people who want to avoid metabolic syndrome or who have metabolic syndrome and want to reverse it. The program is based on critical factors that can get you healthy for life. We have carefully considered hundreds of programs and activities and have found five key factors that are essential to health and longevity. These five factors are all you need to remarkably change your life, because they will get you to eat better, move better and think better. The five critical factors of 8 Weeks to Wellness® are:

- Chiropractic Care
- Exercise
- Nutrition
- Mindful Based Stress Reduction
- Massage

We will discuss each one of these aspects in detail in the following chapters.

13

8WW Success Story

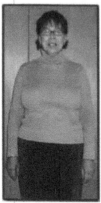

Lost 17 Pounds!
Body Fat
Before: 39% *After:* 35%
Lost 2.5 inches off waist
Lost 2.0 inches off hips

Health Satisfaction:
Before: 52 points,
After: 116 points

Alice Higgins

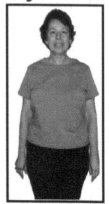

Before   **After**

Where do I begin to thank you and the entire staff of the 8 Weeks to Wellness program? In the fall of 2005 I was going to have some repair work done on my engagement and wedding rings. I had been waiting some time as the repair was a bit pricey, but my husband and I were coming up on a big anniversary and I thought it would be worth it.

At the same time, I was watching my neighbor melt away and feel so good about herself. When I asked her what she was doing, she told me about the 8 Weeks to Wellness program. So after listening to her enthusiasm I thought, "The heck with my wedding rings, I'm going to do some repair work on myself."

I was beginning to have trouble just opening my car door because of my rheumatoid arthritis. I always had a theory that I want to live until I die. But I wasn't doing that. And although I know the best way to live until I die is a healthy lifestyle, I had really slipped. Then came the 8 Weeks to Wellness program.

I chose to do the 8WW program in December of 2005. For most people this would have been a difficult time, but I was determined not to gain the usual 10 pounds over the holidays.

(continued on next page)

8WWW Success Story

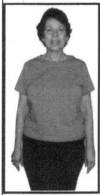

After

Lost 17 Pounds!
Body Fat
Before: 39% *After:* 35%
Lost 2.5 inches off waist
Lost 2.0 inches off hips

Health Satisfaction:
Before: 52 points,
After: 116 points

Alice Higgins

(continued from previous page)

I accomplished this and much, much more. Not only did I NOT gain the usual 10 pounds, but I lost 17 pounds over the 8 week program. Although I didn't love exercise, coming to the office and feeling the love and support of the entire staff, made it so much more fun. The chiropractic care, the massage, all the elements of the program were like small gifts I gave myself.

It's been one month since I completed the program, and I continue to perform all the elements of the program that I was taught. My blood pressure is normal. All my blood work is within normal range. My clothes actually fit. I just simply feel good. I feel confident that I will now LIVE until I die.

A very heartfelt and sincere thank you to you all.

8WᵂW Success Story

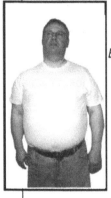

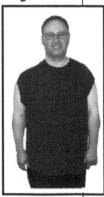

Lost 39 Pounds!
Body Fat
Before: 44.1% *After:* 37.2%
BP Diastolic
from 90 to 70
Glucose
From 125 to 95
Triglycerides/HDL Ratio
from 6.36 to 2.37
Health Satisfaction:
Before: 65 points,
After: 140 points

Before

After

Jim

In July of 2008, I went to my doctor and she advised me to work on getting my weight down. I have a family history of diabetes. It led to my father's death and has been troublesome to some of his brothers and sisters.

On my way back to work I saw the sign for 8 Weeks to Wellness and decided to give them a call. I liked what I heard so I set up an appointment. I came in for the initial visit and signed up to come to a "WOW" presentation.

It was several months before I actually came back to start the 8 Weeks to Wellness program, but little by little I started to make some of the changes recommended in the presentation. I stopped drinking diet soda, paid better attention to what I was eating and avoided high fructose corn syrup and partially hydrogenated oils.

I was making excuse after excuse to avoid signing up; vacation, a big project at work, and the Phillies making the playoffs. By the time I scheduled my appointment for Nov. 3rd, the Phillies playoff run was in full swing and I was ready to make some changes in my life.

(continued on next page)

8WTW Success Story

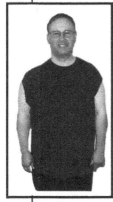

After

Lost 39 Pounds!
Body Fat
Before: 44.1% *After:* 37.2%
BP Diastolic
from 90 to 70
Glucose
From 125 to 95
Triglycerides/HDL Ratio
from 6.36 to 2.37
Health Satisfaction:
Before: 65 points,
After: 140 points

Jim

(continued from previous page)

I lost 10 pounds on my own, and finished the 8 Weeks to Wellness program losing another 29 pounds. I've lost a total loss of 39 pounds. More importantly, my blood sugar level has fallen 30 points since July and I am no longer a high-risk candidate for diabetes!

I owe a BIG thank you to the trainers at 8 Weeks to Wellness, who are always willing to push me and come up with different activities to keep the work-outs interesting. I am also thankful for everyone at the office for their encouragement, good wishes and hard work. Without that, I don't think my success could have been possible.

Sources:

1. *Centers for Disease Control and Prevention.* Centers for Disease Control and Prevention, 11 Jan. 2013.

2. Lakka H, Laaksonen DE, Lakka TA, et al. The Metabolic Syndrome and Total and Cardiovascular Disease Mortality in Middle-aged Men. JAMA. 2002;288(21):2709-2716. doi:10.1001/jama.288.21.2709.

3. Ervin, R. Bethene, Ph.D., R.D.. "Prevalence of Metabolic Syndrome Among Adults 20 Years of Age and Over, by Sex, Age, Race and Ethnicity, and Body Mass Index: United States, 2003–2006." *National Health Statistics Reports.* Centers for Disease Control and Prevention, 5 May 2009. Web.

4. http://www.medicinenet.com/insulin_resistance/article.htm#insulin_resistance_facts.

5. "Type 1 Diabetes Facts - JDRF." 2013. 22 Dec. 2013 http://jdrf.org/about-jdrf/fact-sheets/type-1-diabetes-facts/.

6. "Type 2 - American Diabetes Association®." 2009. 22 Dec. 2013 <http://www.diabetes.org/diabetes-basics/type-2/.

7. Rewers, M. "Why Do People With Diabetes Die Too Soon? - Diabetes Care." 2008.

8. "National Diabetes Statistics, 2011 - National Diabetes Information ..." 2004. 22 Dec. 2013 http://diabetes.niddk.nih.gov/dm/pubs/statistics/.

9. "Body Fat Types (Brown, White, Visceral) and Locations (Belly, Butt ..." 2009. 22 Dec. 2013 http://www.webmd.com/diet/features/the-truth-about-fat?page=2.

10. Alberti, KGMM et al. "Harmonizing the Metabolic Syndrome A Joint Interim Statement of the International Diabetes Federation Task Force on Epidemiology and Prevention; National Heart, Lung, and Blood Institute; American Heart Association; World Heart Federation; International Atherosclerosis Society; and International Association for the Study of Obesity." Circulation 120.16 (2009): 1640-1645.

11. "High Triglycerides: Causes, Treatment, and How to Lower ... - WebMD." 2007. 22 Dec. 2013 <http://www.webmd.com/cholesterol-management/tc/high-triglycerides-overview.

12. "Good vs. Bad Cholesterol - American Heart Association." 2010. 22 Dec. 2013 http://www.heart.org/HEARTORG/Conditions/Cholesterol/A boutCholesterol/Good-vs-Bad-Cholesterol_UCM_305561_Article.jsp.

13. "Good vs. Bad Cholesterol - American Heart Association." 2010. 22 Dec. 2013 <http://www.heart.org/HEARTORG/Conditions/Cholesterol/ AboutCholesterol/Good-vs-Bad-Cholesterol_UCM_305561_Article.jsp>.

14. "Cholesterol HDL/LDL/Triglycerides Ratios Calculator - HughChou.org." 2010. 22 Dec. 2013 http://www.hughchou.org/calc/chol.php.

15. "Glucose test - blood: MedlinePlus Medical Encyclopedia." 2002. 22 Dec. 2013 <http://www.nlm.nih.gov/medlineplus/ency/article/003482.htm.

16. "EPIC - European Prospective Investigation into Cancer and Nutrition." 2008. 22 Dec. 2013 http://epic.iarc.fr/.

17. "High Blood Pressure and Smoking: Risks and Effects." WebMD. WebMD.

18. "Calculate Your BMI - National Heart, Lung, and Blood Institute." 2013. 22 Dec. 2013 http://www.nhlbi.nih.gov/guidelines/obesity/BMI/bmicalc.htm.

2

Chiropractic Care

"The master of your body did not run off and leave you masterless." ~B.J. Palmer

Your brain and spine are the major part of your nervous system and through it control every part of your body.[1]

This includes how you move, how your organs function, your senses (hearing, vision, smell, touch and taste), your immune system and more. In order to be healthy, your nerves, spinal cord and brain must be able to communicate with each other without interference. When there is an ailment, a discomfort, a disease or any medical condition, there is usually a problem with this communication.

Consider you are on the phone getting directions to a location. If there is static on the line when getting your instructions you may not hear them accurately, or you may not hear them at all. Can you hear me now? Let me say it again, so you understand because this is the important part: If there is a problem with the line of communication between your spine and your brain, your brain may not be getting the correct message from the body or be able to direct the body the way it was designed. If this happens you are likely to experience illness, discomfort or dis-ease. Chiropractic clears the obstacles that interrupt this communication. Chiropractors repair the communication so the signals can be properly received again.

Chiropractic is concerned with the preservation and restoration of health, and focuses particular attention on the subluxation. A subluxation is a complex of functional and/or pathological articular changes that compromise neural integrity and may influence organ system function and general health.[2]

The field of chiropractic care began in 1895 by a man named Daniel David Palmer, referred to as D.D. Palmer.[3] He is known as the founder of chiropractic and actually named the treatment with the help of a friend, Rev. Samuel

Weed[4,] when they combined the two words cheiros and prakitkos, which together mean, "done by hand"[5.] When Palmer restored hearing to Harvey Lillard[6], after noticing a bone that appeared displaced on his back, Palmer said, "I reasoned that if that vertebra was replaced, the man's hearing should be restored." After this initial discovery D.D. Palmer, who had already been a teacher and a magnetic healer[7], began to treat people who would seek his help for a variety of ailments. Palmer's work with correcting the spine to affect the healing and health of the body caused him to resume studying anatomy and physiology. In 1898, he transformed his clinic into a school and began teaching the principles and practice of chiropractic.[8] His son, BJ Palmer, went on to develop the field of chiropractic after he took control of the school, now known as Palmer College[9], and began promoting chiropractic treatment as a health profession.

Because chiropractors work with the spine, chiropractic care is often thought of as a treatment for neck and back pain but it is actually aimed more at addressing the cause of problems rather than the effects of them, such as pain. The chiropractic lifestyle more broadly defined is a way of describing a healthy way of living. This includes nutrition, exercise and keeping the body running at optimal levels so it can maintain perfect health. We like to note the difference between *Chiropractic Care* (the adjustment of the spine to correct misalignments that affect the nervous system) and *the Care of a Chiropractor*, which may include instruction and guidance on how to address the underlying problems in your lifestyle that may have created the symptomatic problem with which you are suffering. After all, the word "Doctor" means "Teacher" in Latin.[10]

The body is a self-healing organism. When it is free of interference and given all of the necessary requirements for proper function, such as good nutrition, water, sunlight, etc., it will remain healthy. When the interference to proper function is removed it will get healthy.

Our body works by sending and receiving signals from the brain to the body through the nervous system. In fact, "90% of the stimulation and nutrition to the brain is generated by the movement of the spine," explains Dr. Roger Sperry, Nobel Prize Recipient for Brain Research.

These signals travel from the brain down the spinal cord and out through spinal openings, and through these nerves to every organ, tissue and cell of your body. These signals also run in the opposite direction, from the cells and tissues all the way back to the brain. In fact, there are many more signals going *to* your brain than *from* your brain. This creates an ongoing feedback loop. It allows us to respond to temperature, visual stimuli, sounds, smells, recently eaten foods and body positions, as well as to enable us to handle foreign invaders such as bacteria and viruses and many other environmental stimuli.

If our body and brain need to communicate in order to function properly, then what are the obstacles that can get in the way? The answer is misalignment of the spine, known as subluxations.[11] Vertebral subluxations (see figure A below) are when a bone in your spine is misaligned, moving improperly, or out of place. This is what creates that "static" in the communication, and a chiropractic adjustment is the art of adjusting the bone to allow it to move better, thereby clearing away the obstacle and allowing the signals to get through.

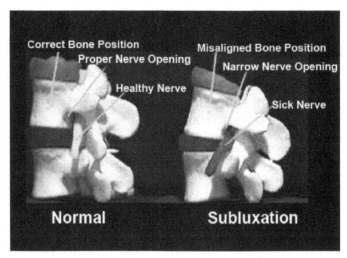

Figure A

Subluxations are caused by stress. Stress comes in three basic forms: chemical, emotional and physical.[12]

Chemical Stress

Chemical stress includes the bad foods we eat, the medications we take and the environment in which we live. Even if you exercise, get enough sleep and have great relationships, if you don't eat right you will not be healthy. This lack of health not only comes from the weight gain of not eating correctly, but also from the subluxations caused by the chemical stress. We see this often in our patients on Monday mornings, after a late night football game enjoyed with chicken wings and beer for dinner. That is not what the body needs to keep healthy!

Emotional Stress

Emotional stress comes from bad relationships, an unhappy work environment and an unhealthy mental attitude. Tense relationships with ourselves, our spouse, our children and even our money can cause emotional stress that can lead to subluxations, sickness and disease. We see this most in our patients when they are going through a divorce, having financial difficulties or even around the holidays. Why do people get sick during or after holidays? It's often the most emotionally stressful time of the year. More frequent chiropractic adjustments are needed during the emotionally stressed times of our lives.

Physical Stress

Physical stress is the stress most people think about when they think about their spines. We find that the subluxations caused by physical stress usually have some underlying chemical or emotional component to go along with them. How can two people involved in the same car accident have two totally different injuries? Usually it has to do with the stresses the people had on their systems immediately prior to the accident. Physical stress includes accidents, slips and falls, poor lifting techniques and even pregnancy. Physical stress can be caused by trauma, but it can also be caused by lifestyle conditions and habits. What most people don't consider is that poor posture, long flights, bad beds, improper use of pillows, being overweight, improper exercise, recliners and a sedentary lifestyle all are elements of physical stress.

There are signs that your body is not dealing well with stress.[13]

Emotional symptoms of stress include:

- Becoming easily agitated, frustrated, and moody
- Feeling overwhelmed, as if you are losing control or need to take control
- Having difficulty relaxing and quieting your mind
- Feeling badly about yourself (low self-esteem)
- Feeling lonely, worthless and depressed
- Avoiding others

Physical symptoms of stress include:

- Low energy
- Headaches
- Upset stomach, including diarrhea, constipation, and nausea
- Aches, pains, and tense muscles
- Chest pain and rapid heartbeat
- Insomnia
- Frequent colds and infections
- Loss of sexual desire and/or ability
- Nervousness and shaking
- Ringing in the ears
- Cold or sweaty hands and feet
- Dry mouth and difficulty swallowing
- Clenched jaw and grinding teeth

Cognitive symptoms of stress include:

- Constant worrying
- Racing thoughts
- Forgetfulness and disorganization
- Inability to focus
- Poor judgment
- Being pessimistic or seeing only the negative side

Behavioral symptoms of stress include:

- Changes in appetite -- either not eating or eating too much
- Procrastinating and avoiding responsibilities
- Increased use of alcohol, drugs, or cigarettes
- Exhibiting more nervous behaviors, such as nail biting, fidgeting and pacing

There are many additional disruptions to your body as well.

Chiropractors have extensive education in anatomy and physiology and are trained to diagnose and treat the various conditions that cause problems. Subluxations are common and unavoidable. Remember, common does not mean normal. Much like cavities, it's not whether we get them in our lives, but when. There is a big difference between "common" and "normal." Subluxations, much like cavities, are common but they are far from normal. Subluxations are common because our bodies undergo physical, chemical and emotional stresses every day and all of these contribute to subluxations. Any of these can possibly affect the nervous system and the improper communication in our nervous system can cause our spine to come out of alignment. When our body is not in alignment it can cause strain on the body, creating tension in the nervous system and eventually pain, illness or disease. *Distortion in the spine and nervous system creates strain on the spine and nervous system.*

We prefer to have the body working at 100% of its potential and no less. This is like when the front end of our car is out of alignment, it creates strain on one part of the tire, causing the whole tire to wear unevenly and thus the tire becomes "worn out" earlier than it should. Not to mention the car will not perform as well as it could. You can still drive it, but it will not be as responsive, track as well, get as good gas mileage, last as long or corner as well as it should. Most people spend too much of their life out of alignment and, like the car, this causes a multitude of performance problems. Because of the loading of gravity and the weight of our bodies, our bodies crave alignment and symmetry. When our body is aligned we are strain-free, stronger and our body functions more effortlessly and is more able to prevent disease and illness.

Let's turn our attention to one of the most common subluxation patterns chiropractors see and treat on a regular basis. It's called "Forward Head Posture"[14] and it is a subluxation of the lower cervical and upper thoracic vertebrae (base of your neck). Seen below in figure A, forward head posture occurs when the vertebrae of the spine subluxate in such a way that the head starts to move forward out in front of the shoulders and hips. When this happens, the neck is burdened with the challenging task of supporting and moving the human head. In fact, Rene Cailliet, M.D., a famous medical author and former director of the department of physical medicine and rehabilitation at the University of Southern California, states:

"Head in forward posture can add up to thirty pounds of abnormal leverage on the cervical spine. This can pull the entire spine out of alignment. Forward head posture (FHP) may result in the loss of 30% of vital lung capacity. These breath-related effects are primarily due to the loss of the cervical lordosis, which blocks the action of the hyoid muscles, especially the inferior hyoid responsible for helping lift the first rib during inhalation."[15]

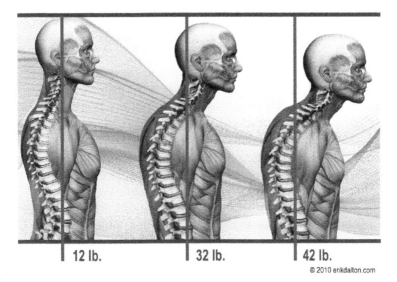

12 lb.   32 lb.   42 lb.

© 2010 erikdalton.com

Figure B

The consequences of subluxation are alarming. In the journal of the *American Geriatric Society*, published in 2004, it shows that if you have forward head posture there was a greater risk of death. In cause-specific mortality analyses, hyperkyphotic posture was specifically associated with an increased rate of death due to atherosclerosis.[16]

Correction of this subluxation pattern and neck posture is key to stopping and reversing degenerative arthritis and pain that causes headaches, rib dysfunction, TMJ and the unattractive Dowager's Humps (the physical deformity that happens as we get a hump in our upper back as noted in figure B above).

English philosopher Bertrand Russell once stated, "A physical system expresses its energy (ability to do work) through function (movement)." Any loss of function sets off reactions within the body, which manifests as structural abnormalities (subluxation and misalignment).

It is common to have subluxations and be unaware of it. This is because they start off subtly with minimal discomfort or pain. That is why it's important to be checked by your chiropractor to see if you need an adjustment.

Your body is your most prized possession. If you think of it the way you'd think of having a sports car like a Ferrari, consider treating it with the same concern. Would you put inferior fuel into your Ferrari? Not likely. So don't put inferior fuel into your body and instead, feed it the best nutrients. Would you service your Ferrari only when it broke down? If so, you will wind up with costly repairs and possibly permanent damage. So instead, you take the car in for its regularly scheduled checkups to ensure you can prevent any problems. That is the same way you should treat your body, keeping it fine tuned so that you can prevent illness and disease. That's what chiropractic care is about.

When you begin to feel the impact of a subluxation it has often been there a long time and shows up as:

- Headaches
- Backaches
- Neck pain
- Joint pain
- Insomnia
- Muscle spasms
- Fatigue
- Colds
- Allergies
- Carpal Tunnel

- Bursitis
- Asthma
- Heart or chest conditions
- Anemia
- Heartburn or indigestion
- Cramps
- Constipation
- Sciatica
- Poor circulation
- Tingling or numbness
- Hemorrhoids
- Earache
- And much more

Unfortunately these symptoms often cause people to seek traditional medical care, which can provide relief in the way of drugs and surgery. Traditional medicine is the art of providing symptomatic relief for an ailment. Our health care system today is actually a sick care system, because conventional medicine is sought most often to fix or decrease the symptom through drugs and surgery as opposed to correcting the cause of the problem.

Chiropractic care, on the other hand, is a health profession that traces the symptom back to the cause. For example, someone suffering with a headache may have a subluxation at C1, also called the atlas (the bone in the upper neck). An adjustment to realign this bone can eliminate the headache. Or, someone who has asthma or trouble breathing could have a misalignment at T1 (the bone and nerve associated with the arms, elbows, hands, wrists, fingers, esophagus and trachea). Traditional medical care would provide drugs (some for long-term usage) to clear up the symptoms or effect but if the cause of the symptom is not corrected, the symptom will reoccur.

Chiropractic care is the art of adjusting the spine and extremities of the body. A chiropractors care is the art of helping people get and maintain a healthy body. It encompasses more than just adjusting the spine and extremities. The chiropractic lifestyle includes nutrition, exercise, a positive attitude and helping the body function at its optimal level.

Health and well-being truly occur from the inside-out, not from the outside-in. As a matter of fact, because of the unhealthy environment that we've created in the past 100 years, we've gotten to the point where we need *two* primary care doctors, a "Sickcare Doctor," the doctor we see when we are sick, and a "Healthcare Doctor," the doctor we see to keep from getting sick."

Almost everyone knows who their "Sickcare Doctor" is, it's the primary care physician we go to (usually an MD) when we are sick. However, the right chiropractor needs to be viewed as your true "Healthcare Doctor," the doctor we see to stay healthy **regardless of symptoms**. The more time and energy you invest into staying healthy, the less you will need to invest in dealing with sickness.

And What About Our Children?

When is the best time to start chiropractic care? We suggest that it is important to have a proper functioning nervous system from the womb to the tomb. As chiropractors, we have adjusted our own children since they were born. Our children average less than two sick days a year and have never had the ongoing rounds of antibiotics, asthma and allergy meds, ADHD meds, etc. that we see in most American children. Coincidence? We think not. In our chiropractic offices we see newborns and infants regularly. The great thing is that they require very little care as they do not have the stress that adults have. An adjustment to a subluxated two year olds' nervous system can change the rest of their life.

Testimonial

My six-year-old daughter has been dealing with constipation since she was born. The very first instance was when she was three months old. Since then, we have been to several doctors. They all did the same tests, and prescribed the same medications; stool softeners, fiber laxatives and others. All of these helped to some degree, but nothing was able to fully relieve her upset stomach and constant constipation.

When she was five, she started to have traces of blood in her bowel movements. I took her to the doctor again. He x-rayed her stomach and prescribed over the counter laxatives. That evening, I was in to see my chiropractor for a regular visit. He asked me why I was so tense that day and I told him about my daughter's problem. He asked me to bring her in with me at my appointment; he might be able to help her. I didn't really believe there was anything he could do, but I was desperate to find something to help her.

At that appointment, he examined her spine and adjusted her lower back. He explained to me that there is a nerve that controls the bowels, and if that nerve is pinched, it creates bowel problems. From that day and for the next two weeks, my daughter had a bowel movement every day.

That was five months ago. Since then, with regular adjustments, my daughter no longer complains of an upset stomach. The blood has disappeared from her stool and she is much more regular. A child who used to come home from school and lay on the couch in front of the TV because her stomach hurt, now begs to go outside and play, no matter what the weather is.

There are many people who are skeptical about chiropractic care. I was one of those skeptics. I didn't understand how important something as simple as proper adjustment was to a person's total health and well-being. I am thankful that my chiropractor was able to help my daughter and save her from possible life-long discomfort.

- LH.

Research on children and chiropractic can be found at icpa4kids.org. There you can find many articles detailing how chiropractic benefits all types of conditions including:[17]

- Abdominal Pain - (1 Article)
- Acid Reflux (Gerd) - (1 Article)
- Attention Deficit Disorder/ADHD - (12 Articles)
- Asthma - (22 Articles)
- Ataxia, Dizziness and Visual Disturbance
  - (1 Article)
- Autism, Behavioral and Learning Disorders
  - (15 Articles)
- Bed Wetting - (10 Articles)
- Bell's Palsy - (7 Articles)
- Birth Abnormalities - (1 Article)
- Birth Trauma - (2 Articles)

- Blindness - (1 Article)
- Blood Pressure/Hypertension - (12 Articles)
- Brain Function/Emotional Health - (26 Articles)
- Breastfeeding Difficulties - (9 Articles)
- Carpal Tunnel Syndrome - (16 Articles)
- Cerebral Palsy - (2 Articles)
- Childhood Diseases - (2 Articles)
- Chiropractic: Efficacy, Safety and Satisfaction - (18 Articles)
- Colic - (14 Articles)
- Common Cold - (6 Articles)
- Constipation - (3 Articles)
- Crib Death (SIDS) - (7 Articles)
- Crohn's Disease/Colitis - (3 Articles)
- Ear Infection (Otitis Media) - (25 Articles)
- Epilepsy/Seizures - (11 Articles)
- Erb's Palsy - (4 Articles)
- Facial Symmetry - (1 Article)
- Female Concerns - (5 Articles)
- Fever - (2 Articles)
- Growing Pains - (1 Article)
- Headaches /Migraine - (26 Articles)
- Immune Function - (13 Articles)
- Infertility/Inability to Conceive - (12 Articles)
- Injury - (4 Articles)
- Mind, Body, Spirit - (1 Article)
- Motor Tics - (1 Article)
- Neck Pain (5 Articles)
- Pediatric Care - (2 Articles)
- Pregnancy and Adjustments - (12 Articles)
- Quality of Life/Wellness - (15 Articles)
- Respiratory Function and Breathing Ability - (19 Articles)
- Satisfaction, Cost, and Safety of Chiropractic
- - (21 Articles)
- Scoliosis - (10 Articles)

- Sinus and Respiratory Infections/Sinusitis
  - (5 Articles)
- Skin/Eczema/Psoriasis - (3 Articles)
- Sleep - (3 Articles)
- Speech Disorders - (3 Articles)
- Spinal Health - (7 Articles)
- Sports Performance and Chiropractic - (4 Articles)
- Stuttering - (1 Article)
- Thyroid - (4 Articles)
- TMJ Syndrome, Dental Health - (6 Articles)
- Tonsillitis - (5 Articles)
- Torticollis - (13 Articles)
- Tourette's Syndrome - (2 Articles)
- Tremors - (1 Article)
- Vision Problems - (4 Articles)
- Webster Technique - (7 Articles)

We do not want to just correct subluxations, we want to prevent them through a chiropractic lifestyle! As a true healthcare chiropractor, we are full-scope *Chiropractic Physicians* versus chiropractors who are limited scope and only treat pain. If, as doctors, we only treated the disease of subluxations we would only be doing part of the job. This would be like a dentist only fixing cavities, without cleaning the teeth, promoting dental hygiene and preventing tooth decay. Why keep bailing water out of the boat when you could plug the hole? Better yet, keep your boat healthy so it never gets holes! A program like 8 Weeks to Wellness® is the way to prevent subluxations! That is why we are so passionate about the program. It addresses the physical, chemical and emotional causes of subluxation.

And the chiropractic aspect of the 8 Weeks to Wellness® program keeps your body communicating clearly.

8WW Success Story

"I lost over 30 pounds!"

Amy Harvey, M.D.

As a physician I have counseled many of my patients on the need for weight loss and maintenance of a healthy lifestyle. However, for over two decades I myself struggled with my own weight issue. Approximately six months ago I had the pleasure of visiting with some of my own patients who had participated in your "8 Weeks to Wellness" program. I was amazed and delighted to see how healthy, energetic, and toned they had become. They all spoke highly of you, your staff, and your program. As you know, I have tried numerous diet plans without success and I was addicted to my sedentary lifestyle. Your program appeared to be a fine balance of nutritional support, mindful eating, and physical activity including both cardiovascular and strength-training exercises; all with an emphasis on self-nurturing. What an amazing concept!!

Having been through my eight weeks and then some, I must say your program was everything you said and even more! I have now lost over 30 pounds and have dropped my fasting glucose levels more than 30 points. The difference in my energy is unbelievable. As you know, I live a fairly busy lifestyle and I truly enjoy the time I make for myself when it comes to visiting you and your staff. I must make a special comment regarding your staff at the Center. They really make the program so infectious. They are motivating, encouraging, positive, and they all truly love their jobs. That is a true testimonial to your brilliant work.

(continued on next page)

8WWW Success Story

"I lost over 30 pounds!"

Amy Harvey, M.D.

(continued from previous page)

I consider your "8 Weeks to Wellness" program to be one of the greatest gifts I have ever given myself. And, for this, I thank you. I am now a role model to my patients, staff, colleagues, and friends; and I am living proof that a life of balance with healthy eating and a well-planned exercise regimen is still the only way to true wellness. Plus, all of the positive feedback I receive from those who remember the "old me" is just the icing on the cake!!! Thank you for getting me back on track and for showing me the path to the new and improved me! I am delighted to have such a terrific place to refer my patients to help them achieve their very own healthy lifestyle, too!

Thank you, for sharing your amazing talents with my patients and me.

8WW Success Story

"I lost over 17 pounds!"
David Garcia

Thank you for sharing your time, energy, and 8 Weeks to Wellness Challenge Program with me. I began the program weighing 184 pounds. I finished the program weighing 166.5 pounds. Both my waist and hip measurements decreased as well. While those changes in numbers I am proud of, I want you to know about the most important transformation.

Growing up, I had a relatively healthy childhood without any major events occurring, until I was 18. That summer I woke up one day with a severe pain that I had never experienced before in my life. The pain was located in my lower back and hips, and it was so intense that I could not walk for periods of time. For 15 years that area would continue to flare up, causing me pain that would last a few days, a few weeks, or too often, several months. I went to every doctor imaginable. They had me take every test imaginable, and still no relief was found. The stiffness, soreness, and pain in that area was daily for 15 years. About 2 years ago I was diagnosed with an autoimmune disease called Ankylosing Spondylitis. It is as bad as it sounds. About a year ago I "accepted" the diagnosis and began infusions of a drug called Remicade (essentially a protein taking from rats to help my body defend itself from itself), and an NSAID. The two never truly gave me complete relief from my symptoms.

(continued on next page)

8WW Success Story

"I lost over 17 pounds!"
David Garcia

(continued from previous page)

I apologize for the long story, but 15 years of going through life in such horrific pain was awful. I began the 8WW program thinking that maybe I could lose a little weight and hopefully feel fitter. I learned immediately that your program was a blessing. I was feeling so good that after 3 weeks I decided to stop the NSAID and suspend my infusions indefinitely. During the 8 weeks that I was following your program, I woke up every morning but three pain and stiffness free. I feel better today than I have felt in 15 years!

When I learned about my colleague's husband willing to share a wellness program at the place where I work, I had no idea what it was. I even considered not doing it. In fact, I did not sign up until the weekend before your introduction.

One of the most meaningful parts of the manual for me was writing down why I wanted to complete the 8WW. My "Why's" for doing the program included me wanting to grow old with my wife and be healthy in order to enjoy our time together, me having energy to help my children grow up to be great people, and me being pain free. Because of 8WW, I believe that today I am living my "Why's" and I have God to thank for putting me in the right place at the right time to accept the 8WW Challenge.

I also have to thank you, for having integrity, compassion, unselfishness, and kindness. You shared your life's work with me. In doing so, you helped changed my life forever. I am forever indebted to you.

With Great Admiration and Appreciation.

Sources:

1. "Nervous System Information - Penn Medicine." 2009.
27 Dec. 2013
<http://www.pennmedicine.org/health_info/body_guide/reft
ext/html/nerv_sys_fin.html>
"Chiropractic care for children: Controversies and issues."
2010. 29.

2. "Chiropractic care for children: Controversies and
issues." 2010. 29 Dec. 2013
http://www.ncbi.nlm.nih.gov/pmc/articles/PMC2794701/.

3. "The Palmer Family - Palmer College of Chiropractic."
2011. 27 Dec. 2013
http://www.palmer.edu/ThePalmerFamily/.

4. "Palmer Green Books - Palmer College of Chiropractic."
2011. 27 Dec. 2013
<http://www.palmer.edu/PalmerGreenBooks/>.

5. PALMER, BJ. "Science of Chiropractic." 1906.
http://www.therscproject.com/wp-
content/uploads/2011/05/The-Science-of-Chiropractic-Its-
Principles-and-Philosophies-1920.pdf.

6. "Harvey Lillard - Palmer College of Chiropractic." 2012.
29 Dec. 2013
http://www.palmer.edu/020112africanamericanhistory/.

7. "D.D. Palmer's Lifeline - Chiro.Org." 2006. 29 Dec. 2013
http://www.chiro.org/Plus/History/Persons/PalmerDD/Palm
erDD's-Lifeline-chrono.pdf.

8. Batinić, J. "Did American social and economic events from 1865 to 1898 ..." 2013. http://www.ncbi.nlm.nih.gov/pmc/articles/PMC3743648/.

9. "Our History - Palmer College of Chiropractic." 2010. 29 Dec. 2013 http://www.palmer.edu/history/.

10. "Doctor - Definition and More from the Free Merriam-Webster Dictionary." 2005. 29 Dec. 2013 http://www.merriam-webster.com/dictionary/doctor.

11. "subluxation - definition of subluxation in the Medical dictionary - by ..." 2005. 29 Dec. 2013 http://medical-dictionary.thefreedictionary.com/subluxation.

12. "3 Types of Stress | - Fit to Live." 2013. 29 Dec. 2013 http://fittolivetoday.com/blog/3-types-of-stress/.

13 "Stress Symptoms: Effects of Stress on the Body - WebMD." 2011. 29 Dec. 2013 http://www.webmd.com/balance/stress-management/stress-symptoms-effects_of-stress-on-the-body.

14. "FORWARD HEAD POSTURE - Chiro.Org." 2006. 29 Dec. 2013 http://www.chiro.org/LINKS/Forward_Head_Posture.shtml.

15. "FORWARD HEAD POSTURE - Chiro.Org." 2006. 29 Dec. 2013 http://www.chiro.org/LINKS/Forward_Head_Posture.shtml.

16. Kado, Deborah M et al. "Hyperkyphotic Posture Predicts Mortality in Older Community-Dwelling Men and Women: A Prospective Study." Journal of the American Geriatrics Society 52.10 (2004): 1662-1667.

17. "ICPA - Public Wellness Education and Chiropractic Research." 2004. 29 Dec. 2013 http://icpa4kids.org/.

3

Exercise

Lack of activity destroys the good condition of every human being, while movement and methodical physical exercise save it and preserve it. ~Plato

How Important Is Exercise?

You were born to move! As humans, we were made to play when we are young and to work physically when we became adults. That is how we got our food, water and shelter, protected our homes and countries and provided a living for a family. That is how we are designed and it worked well over the time man has been on planet Earth, until something changed. What changed is that people no longer *have* to move to survive. You can literally never work up a sweat from the day you are born till the day you die with today's modern conveniences. This is not how you were designed to function. It is like asking a fish to climb a tree and then judging the fish on his ability to climb that tree. You would call the fish a failure, just as we would call most people's health a failure when they are not moving sufficiently. You were not designed to be sedentary any more than a fish was designed to climb a tree.

However, many people actually do live a sedentary lifestyle and yet desire to be healthy, or even fit. It is simply not possible. If you eat well but never exercise, you may have normal weight but no muscle mass. This can cause you to be what we call skinny fat. Many vegetarians fall into this category because of their high carbohydrate consumption and lack of intense physical activity.

Exercise is essential. In fact, your body can deal better with a few poor food choices than if you only ate healthy foods but never exercised. Exercising your body makes it work more efficiently, as well as providing a host of other benefits. Without exercise, regardless of your diet, you decrease your health, because your body is losing muscle mass and flexibility. Moreover, we know that the "ultimate stiffness" is called death and nobody should want to move faster towards it than is already happening!

Many people embark on an exercise program to lose weight or look better. Whatever gets you to exercise is good in itself, but our goal is to get you to exercise for your life. There was a time when our need to exist required exercise. Moving and working physically was necessary or we would die. Hunting for food, traveling by foot, building by hand was a part of life. With modern technology, everything is done for us by others and by remote controls. Obesity and other health-related problems are becoming rampant in our population. In fact, the rates of obesity (36% of us) have skyrocketed in the past 50 years, especially in our children. And the cost of this obesity is killing the U.S. economy. The estimated annual medical cost of obesity in the U.S. was $147 billion in 2008 U.S. dollars; the medical costs for people who are obese were $1,429 higher per year than those of normal weight.[1]

When people begin a physical fitness program for any reason the benefits are many. These benefits include:

- Increased metabolism
- Increased cardiovascular strength
- Increased mental performance
- Improved sleep
- Decreased depression
- Increased energy
- Increased libido
- Decreased risk of most common degenerative diseases
- And many more

If the above benefits came in a pill, would you take it? Of course you would, even if it took an hour to take it! But many people don't exercise. According to the CDC, only 20.6% of Americans get the recommended amount of cardiovascular and strength training exercise per week.[2]

This is not entirely their fault as most of America has not been taught the importance of exercise and how to exercise properly. Gone are the days of daily gym class in our public schools. Our parents were never taught these skills to pass them down because our parents and their parents didn't need to go to the gym to get the required amount of physical activity. They got it because they worked hard physically without having to go to the gym. So how do most Americans learn to exercise? From an infomercial or a videotape?

Unfortunately, because of this we are the most obese people in the world. When you learn to exercise properly the payoffs are huge. When you continue to work properly and consistently your health improves and remains functioning at optimal levels. We want everyone to know how to exercise.... properly.

So how do you get these benefits? In any good wellness program such as the *8 Weeks to Wellness*® program, you should learn how to exercise properly and to gain the maximum benefit of exercise. This doesn't mean you have to work extra hard or extra long. In fact, knowing the proper techniques should give you a more quality workout in less time.

You don't have to use a lot of machines to exercise. In fact, we use exercises that complement life's actions. In our daily life we run, we move things, we pick up children, we swing golf clubs and baseball bats, we sit down and get up, we reach for things. These are the same simple actions where people often get injured because they aren't movements that are done regularly enough, so their body isn't strong, flexible and agile enough. But with regular training, they could be. We have patients who come in walking crooked, in tremendous pain after simply bending over to pick up something light like a pencil. A pencil doesn't weigh that much! This happens because a person is so deconditioned and out of shape that they can't even bend properly. How about the dad who injures his shoulder throwing a football with his son because his shoulder muscles aren't strong and he hasn't "conditioned" himself for this activity because he doesn't do this type of movement on a regular basis?

We have to ask ourselves an important question as we age: *'Am I going to be limited more and more because I am not conditioned to do the things I once could do? Or am I going to start getting conditioned so that I can do the activities that I enjoy throughout the course of my life such as dance, run, jump, throw, etc.?'* Life becomes pretty miserable when we can't move properly, doesn't it?

It's Not Your Fault That You Don't Know How to Exercise

Many people who exercise aren't reaping the benefits because they are "going through the motions" and don't work at their maximum potential. We all know people who spend countless hours at the gym but don't appear to be in shape. If you are exercising correctly, your body will show it. Period. So, let's learn right now what it means to exercise properly.

We know that there are three essential phases to exercise.[3]

- Strength training against resistance
- Cardio training
- Mobility training

Strength Training

Strength training is working the muscles in your body with resistance. Each session you are pushing yourself to reach a level that is difficult. This builds lean muscle and also strengthens bones[4]. You can do this by lifting free weights, using machines, your own body weight and resistance bands. Our focus is on using your own body weight and free weights such as dumbbells and kettlebells. We utilize free weights because you are controlling the action as opposed to the machine controlling the action and plane of motion. We don't live our lives moving only through one plane of motion and so ultimately we should not train on machines that have only one plane of motion. However, we may need to start our exercise and training this way, since controlling the plane of motion gives stability to the exercise and reduces the risk of injuring ourselves. Also, we want and need to train movements and NOT body parts. In traditional "old school" workouts, we just focus on one or two muscle groups (back and biceps or chest and triceps). This should not be the goal for the average American. Although it may make us look good in the mirror, it does not allow us to accomplish the true goal of exercise, which is better functionality and aging through better functional *movement*.

There are many benefits when you use weights for strength training. Functional weight training does the following[5]:

- Increases lean muscle mass
- Strengthens your bones and increases bone density
- Boosts metabolism
- Delays the effects of aging
- Balances your hormones

- Sharpens your attention
- Reduces blood pressure as well as other conditions that can lead to chronic illnesses

When you work out with weights, you are essentially creating small tears in your muscle fibers. This is GOOD, not bad! If you are sore, consider it payment for a job well done, and know that soreness will result in the addition of more lean body mass (muscle) being added to your body. This is what you want to happen. It takes 48 hours for the muscle to repair and rebuild, during which time you will feel some soreness and should not rework the same area. For example, if you strength train your upper body functional movements one day, you should skip weight training or those same movements the next day. When someone wants to workout with weights every day, they should stagger the areas; upper body focus one day, lower body the next. You can also do a full body workout with weights one day and a cardio workout the next day. The third day you could go back to the weight workout. It is fine to have one day every week when you do not perform exercise and let your body rest.

When you build more lean muscle mass your body will burn more calories all the time.[6] Muscle requires energy. We're not talking about bulk (although the same concept applies) we are talking about *lean compact muscle*. There are methods to use for people who desire to bulk up but for the most part working against resistance will tone and shape your body providing definition and firmness. Lean muscle mass does weigh more than fat so if you are skinny fat (high body fat % with a low muscle %), you may see an increase in your weight as you exercise, but because lean muscle is dense you will look thinner, fitter, and younger because your body shape is changing. Remember *the mirror tells the tale more than the scale*. Plus, you'll be able to consume more calories on a daily basis as your body will require more fuel. Muscle burns 5.5 times[7] more calories at rest than fat so bring on the muscle so you can raise your resting metabolic rate. People who have leaner muscle mass burn more calories at rest than people who are "skinny-fat" or worse "fat-fat." It becomes a doom loop as you get fatter; you burn less calories, allowing you to get fatter and the vicious cycle continues. The only way to break this cycle is to start putting muscle on your body!

Here are some examples of exercises that include resistance to build muscle mass.

Upper Body Functional Exercises
1. Push-ups (multiple variations)
2. Pull-ups (multiple variations)
3. Dumbbell Overhead Press
4. Dumbbell or Barbell Bench Press
5. Dumbbell Bicep Curl
6. Bench Dips
7. Bent-Over or Seated Row
8. Dumbbell Shoulder Rotations

Lower Body Functional Exercises
1. Squat (multiple variations)
2. Lunge (multiple variations)
3. Box Step Ups (variable heights)
4. Dead Lift
5. Leg Curl
6. Calf Raises
7. Good Mornings Back Extensions
8. Kettlebell Swing

Core Functional Exercises
1. Planks (front, side and reverse)
2. Sit-ups, Traditional

3. Twisting Crunching - Bicycle Crunch
4. Windshield Wipers
5. V Sit-ups
6. Pelvic Bridge
7. Burpees
8. Cable Rotations (multiple variations)

Cardio Training

Cardio (short for cardiovascular exercise), or aerobic, exercise strengthens your heart, increases blood pressure and circulation as well as increases your metabolism (and your endurance level)[8] When you sufficiently complete an effective cardio workout you will even burn fat and calories for a few hours after the workout. But how do you know if you are exercising effectively? The only way to know is by knowing what your heart rate is and what your target heart rate should be. Never taught this before? We are not surprised.

Cardiovascular exercise speeds up your heart rate to make it work harder and burn more fuel. But you need to know that you are in the correct heart rate range without over straining or under straining your heart and cardiovascular system. There are two main types of cardiovascular workouts that you need to know: *Aerobic* and *Anaerobic*.

Aerobic cardiovascular exercise involves long duration (over three minutes), less effort-intense work where our heart rate usually stays within 60-80% of our maximum heart rate (determined by taking the number 220 and subtracting your age). *Anaerobic exercise*, as you may have guessed, involves shorter duration, and higher effort-intense bursts of exercise where our heart usually stays between 80-100% of our maximum heart rate (220 - your age)[9].

As mentioned earlier, we recommend that everyone perform their workout with a heart rate monitor to track their exact heart rate. Not knowing what your heart rate is when you're exercising is like baking something without knowing what temperature the oven is set to. You don't know what results you'll get because you don't know your effort intensity.

With proper cardiovascular exercise, HIIT training (High Intensity Interval Training), you should aim for working out for at least 20 minutes, and no more than 30 minutes. During a 20 to 30 minute workout session, you increase your heart rate to 60-90% of its maximum working potential for four to five one-minute cycles during the session. Do this type of training three times a week for a total of 60 to 90 minutes per week. See figure A to understand how a 20 minute HIIT Cardio training session would look.

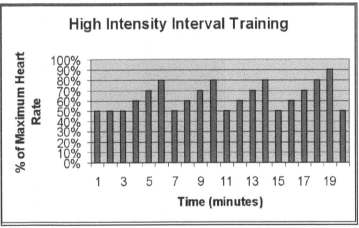

Figure A

How do you figure out your numbers? Your heart rate zone is determined by your age and fitness level. The correct maximum heart rate is the number 220 minus your current age. The range is given to allow for your fitness level.

So remember, *aerobic exercise* is when we say you work at 70–80% of your target heart rate for 30 minutes (see figure B).The 30 minutes *begin* when you reach that percentile. The warm up time to getting there will depend upon your current level of fitness. The more fit you are the longer it may take to get to that level.

Target Heart Rate Maximum Target Training Zones							
	Approximate maximum heart rate	Maximum target training zones (beats per minute)					
Age	Heart rate	60%	65%	70%	75%	80%	85%
20	200	120	130	140	150	160	170
25	195	117	127	137	146	156	166
30	190	114	124	133	143	152	162
35	185	111	120	130	139	148	157
40	180	108	117	126	135	144	153
45	175	105	114	123	131	140	149
50	170	102	111	119	128	136	145
55	165	99	107	116	124	132	140
60	160	96	104	112	120	128	136
65	155	93	101	109	116	124	132
70	150	90	98	105	113	120	128
75	145	87	94	102	109	116	123
80	140	84	91	98	105	112	119

Figure B

In order to check your heart rate, find your pulse on your wrist by placing two fingers on the inside of the wrist about an inch below your thumb. Press lightly until you feel a pulse. Count the heartbeats for 10 seconds and multiply that number by six. That number will tell you what your approximate current heart rate is.[10]

Anaerobic exercise is the HIIT (High Intensity Interval Training) we discussed above. Simply stated, this means you will push hard into the anaerobic zone for brief periods and then lower the intensity to recover. These short interval training session increase your fitness and athletic abilities. It also improves glucose metabolism and fat burning, both of which are required to reduce metabolic syndrome.[11,12,13,14] When performing this type of training, you may wind up doing 30-40 seconds of high intensity work such as an all-out sprint, followed by 60 seconds of recovery such as jogging or walking. Also, remember initially, your all-out sprint may be a jog!

You can see that you don't have to do an hour of aerobics to become aerobically fit. Twenty to 30 minutes will do it when done in the target heart rate zone. When you work out at the correct pace, you will sweat. Sweating is a good sign (as long as you are monitoring your heart rate and not working into a dangerous zone of over 90% of your maximum heart rate).

Is Sweating a Dangerous Sign?

Sweating is actually a good sign. A little sweat plays a big role in keeping you feeling and looking great. It is a sign of work and energy production. Energy, which is defined as the capacity to do work, produces heat and heat in the body causes us to sweat. It literally is a sign of us burning energy, known as calories, in the body. It provides many additional benefits as well.[15] Sweating removes toxins from your body and actually helps keep your skin cleaner. It lowers your body temperature to prevent overheating, which is why it is so important to rehydrate by drinking water when you sweat.

Fitness Training

Mobility/Stability Training

In preparing the body for exercise to receive all the benefits of physical fitness, we include what we call mobility/stability training prior to exercise, which will increase your flexibility, balance and range of motion. Mobility training is often the most overlooked component of exercise and includes exercises like dynamic stretching, which are performed by moving beyond your joints' usual range of motion. In particular, we focus on your core (spinal) mobility and stability. There are 53 joints in your spine and hundreds of muscles that move and stabilize your core. The bottom line is that we simply cannot function properly and have good alignment if we have a weak and inflexible core.

Also called *movement prep*, mobility training is like warming up your car on a cold day before you get in and drive away. Remember, a warm rubber band is going to stretch and bend a lot better than a cold rubber band. In fact, the older we get, the more important this aspect of exercise becomes because the most vulnerable rubber band to breaking is the old, cold rubber band!

Movement prep is done to prepare the body for proper movement where the joints of the body are stable and can move through a good range of motion. When we are tight and our muscles can't elongate, our body has to compensate with abnormal movements. This puts the body in unnatural positions, stressing our muscles and straining our joints. This results in the "bad form" that we regularly see in people who try to exercise without "warming up" properly. Even if people want to use correct form, they can't because their tight muscles and joints won't allow for proper form and movement.

As a matter of fact, a whole new system for evaluating proper movement and function has been developed and is being used extensively with athletes.[16] This is called the "Functional Movement Screen"[17] and it allows the people who use it to see how they are moving and what muscles and joints are preventing proper movement. One very important concept is that we NEVER want to load a dysfunctional movement pattern. In other words, if you can't do the movement properly with just your body's weight, you shouldn't use any more weight such as dumbbells or barbells. For example, we've all seen the guy squatting or benching a lot of weight at the gym, however, if he is not squatting or benching with the right form because he hasn't warmed up his body properly or simply can't perform the movement properly due to misalignment or arthritis, he is actually doing more harm than good in the long term. This is why we don't see many older people at the gym squatting or benching with heavy weights these days. Why? Because they can't. Their tight and worn out muscles and joints won't allow for the weight they once could lift.

We always recommend a movement prep routine at least 10 - 20 minutes three times per week and ideally before your strength training. To learn more about functional movement as opposed to dysfunctional movement (which is what we see most of the time), go to www.functionalmovement.com.

Exercises in this category include things like:

- Hamstring stretching
- Shoulder pass through

- Fire hydrants
- Hip flexor stretching
- Yoga
- Pilates
- Foam rolling

These movements increase your core strength and flexibility and along with proper Chiropractic care, they improve your posture and alignment. These exercises benefit you by lengthening your muscles as well as preventing injuries. They also assist with balance and coordination, which is important to prevent falls as we age.

Ultimately how you move when you're 90 is completely a byproduct and reflection of how you moved (or didn't move) when you were 60, and how you move when you're 60 is a reflection of how you moved (or didn't move) when you were 30. Get it?

We think Isaac Newtown said it best when he said, "An object in motion stays in motion."

8WWW Success Story

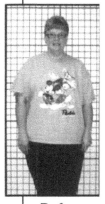

Before

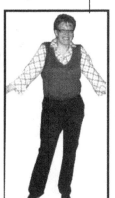

After

Lost 31 Pounds!
Body Fat
Before: 35.8% *After:* 31.5%
Lost 11.5 inches!
Insulin
from 5.7 to 2
Medicial Symptom Score
from 47 to 16

Health Satisfaction:
Before: 78 points,
After: 136 points

Barbara McGarity

My gynecologist, Dr. Amy Harvey, recently informed me of your '8 Weeks to Wellness' program. She suggested in a nice way that I really needed to get more fit due to my various medical problems and weight issue. I left her office in tears. But I went home and discussed the 8WW program with my husband, who said "Give them a call." I did and attended your inspirational 8WW orientation which brought together the entire concept of "wellness" and made a lot of sense to me.

I felt I had everything going against me - very overweight, high blood pressure, Type 2 diabetes, high cholesterol, and a propensity for not exercising. The point in your orientation regarding medications especially hit home.

Now I feel I must write this testimonial to all of you, to your program, your ideals, and your people management skills.

(continued on next page)

8WΨW Success Story

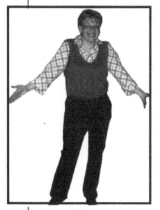

After

Lost 31 Pounds!
<u>Body Fat</u>
Before: 35.8% *After:* 31.5%
Lost 11.5 inches!
Insulin
from 5.7 to 2
Medicial Symptom Score
from 47 to 16

<u>Health Satisfaction:</u>
Before: 78 points,
After: 136 points

Barbara McGarity

(continued from previous page)

To say thank you just doesn't seem enough. Each and every person at your center helped me believe in myself. Because the physical exercise training is the most challenging aspect of fitness, I especially thank you for making me believe I could do it.

I am currently in your "Masters Program" and look forward to working with the 12-week nutritional program next month.

The impact each and every one of you has made on my life goes beyond belief. God bless you all.

8WÆW Success Story

Lost 24 Pounds!
Body Mass Index
Reduced by 3.6 points
Lost 5 inches off waist
Lowered A1c by 1.1%

Earl Pearce

My son and I just completed the 8 Weeks to Wellness program today! Believe me when I tell you IT WORKS! In the last 8 weeks, I have lost 24 pounds, reduced my BMI by 3.6 pts, took 5" off my waistline, lowered my A1c by 1.1% and feel better than I have in years!

I can't say enough about 8 Weeks to Wellness. The entire staff is great, and the program is the real deal! Your knowledge and skills are amazing, but what truly sets your program apart is the genuineness behind it.

EJ and I signed up for a 2nd round of 8 weeks to continue the physical training and conditioning part of the program. Can't stop now!

Sources:

1. "Obesity and Overweight for Professionals: Data and Statistics: Adult ..." 2011. 22 Dec. 2013 http://www.cdc.gov/obesity/data/adult.html.

2. "Press Release - Centers for Disease Control and Prevention." 2013. 29 Dec. 2013 http://www.cdc.gov/media/releases/2013/p0502-physical-activity.html.

3. "Types of Exercise | Exercise Care Guide - Penn Medicine." 2008. 22 Dec. 2013 http://www.pennmedicine.org/health info/exercise/000330. html.

4. "Strength training builds more than muscles - Harvard Health ..." 2012. 22 Dec. 2013 http://www.health.harvard.edu/healthbeat/strength-training-builds-more-than-muscles.

5. Seguin, Rebecca, and Miriam E Nelson. "The benefits of strength training for older adults." American journal of preventive medicine 25.3 (2003): 141-149.

6. "Metabolism and weight loss: How you burn calories - MayoClinic.com." 2005. 22 Dec. 2013 http://www.mayoclinic.com/health/metabolism/WT00006.

7. "How Many Calories Does a Pound of Muscle Burn Per Day ..." 2010. 22 Dec. 2013 http://www.livestrong.com/article/310070-how-many-calories-does-a-pound-of-muscle-burn-per-day/.

8. "Bodybuilding.com - 5 Great Benefits Of Cardiovascular Exercise!." 2007. 22 Dec. 2013 http://www.bodybuilding.com/fun/sclark85.htm.

9. "Target Heart Rates - American Heart Association." 2011. 29 Dec. 2013 http://www.heart.org/HEARTORG/GettingHealthy/Physical Activity/Target-Heart-Rates_UCM_434341_Article.jsp.

10. "Allina Health." How to Check Your Heart Rate. http://www.allinahealth.org/ac/diabetescc.nsf/page/physical _activity_hr.

11. Perry, Christopher GR et al. "High-intensity aerobic interval training increases fat and carbohydrate metabolic capacities in human skeletal muscle." Applied Physiology, Nutrition, and Metabolism 33.6 (2008): 1112-1123.

12. Smith, Abbie E et al. "Effects of β-alanine supplementation and high-intensity interval training on endurance performance and body composition in men; a double-blind trial." Journal of the International Society of Sports Nutrition 6.1 (2009): 1-9.

13. Talanian, Jason L et al. "Two weeks of high-intensity aerobic interval training increases the capacity for fat oxidation during exercise in women." Journal of applied physiology 102.4 (2007): 1439-1447.

14. Talanian, Jason L et al. "Exercise training increases sarcolemmal and mitochondrial fatty acid transport proteins in human skeletal muscle." American Journal of Physiology-Endocrinology And Metabolism 299.2 (2010): E180-E188.

15. "How Sweating Is Good for Your Health - Health - MSN Healthy Living." 2012. 22 Dec. 2013 http://healthyliving.msn.com/health-wellness/how-sweating-is-good-for-your-health-2.

16. Kiesel, Kyle, Phillip J Plisky, and Michael L Voight. "Can serious injury in professional football be predicted by a preseason functional movement screen?." North American journal of sports physical therapy: NAJSPT 2.3 (2007): 147.

17. Cook, Gray. "Movement: Functional Movement Systems." Screening–Assessment–Corrective Strategies. Chichester (UK), Lotuspublishing (2010).

4

Nutrition

"The food you eat can be either the safest and most powerful form of medicine or the slowest form of poison."

~ Ann Wigmore

We've used the car metaphor to describe how to take care of your body a number of times throughout this book. We feel it is a great way to illustrate the type of care your body requires. Think of your body as a complex machine. It takes you places, it protects you, you experience life through the senses it provides. You should care about your body's appearance and its functionality. You will want it to last a long time and not show or be diminished by any wear and tear it encounters over many years of use. You want to keep it running well, and you want to feel good in it.

In order to run well, your car and your body require proper fuel. It may function on lower standards of fuel, but it won't perform as well or last as long that way. So, in this chapter we want to express the importance of fueling your body with the proper nutrients to help you get and maintain a healthy body, and in addition, one that makes you look and feel your best.

Calories Are Not Created Equal

If you think that counting calories is a good way to maintain your weight or help you lose weight, you have been misled like many people. The foods we eat are comprised of a variety of elements that when put together determine whether they can be utilized, broken down and are helpful to our body.

If you required 3,000 calories a day, do you think you'd remain healthy if those 3,000 calories were provided by 30 cans of 100 Calorie Coke? Obviously not. So learning which foods provide the best nourishment for your body is pretty much key to keeping your machine shiny and new, or at least, getting it to provide you with the best protection, the smoothest ride and the finest appearance.

Understanding the Glycemic Index

Glycemic Index:

A system that ranks foods on a scale from 1 to 100 based on their effect on blood-sugar levels.

Our body converts carbohydrates into glucose. The glucose triggers the production of insulin, which takes the sugar out of our bloodstream and draws it into our cells where our body can use it for energy. The Glycemic Index (GI) is a classification index that indicates how your body reacts to the sugar in food. It is a scale to tell us how quickly or how slowly our body will break down sugar.[1] If foods have high sugar content without much fiber it converts to sugar very quickly, sometimes too quickly for our body to use. As we mentioned in our chapter on metabolic syndrome, if we flood our body with sugar too quickly, we stimulate an overabundance of insulin and the body is unable to move the glucose quick enough into the cells. If your diet consistently provides too much glucose, over time the excess insulin it has triggered creates problems. These problems include:

- High triglycerides
- High "bad" LDL cholesterol
- Low "good" HDL cholesterol
- High blood pressure
- Insulin resistance
- Increased appetite
- Obesity
- Risk of type 2 diabetes

If you made the connection, these are the same symptoms in metabolic syndrome. So your diet is one of the key factors to keeping your body healthy. Although an occasional high GI food will not cause significant problems, a consistent diet of them will. In fact, a diet that contains high glycemic foods will also cause you to feel fatigued and hungry because these foods cause insulin to be released in high quantity[2] and this insulin drives the sugar into your cells and then your blood sugar drops. As the saying goes, "that which goes up, must come down." This can stimulate your hunger for even more high glycemic foods. It is a roller coaster effect of spiking your blood sugar and then dropping it.

Your body cannot store carbohydrates and, when your body cannot use the extra sugar for energy it stores it as fat. The goal is to eat foods that break down slowly so there is less fuel converted to fat.

You'll learn how to make your best food choices in the 8WW program, but for now, here's a quick overview of how it works, and why the glycemic index is a valuable tool.

If you are trying to lose weight, control cholesterol, lower triglycerides, reduce the possibilities of diabetes or metabolic syndrome, you want to concentrate on foods that break down slowly. These are foods with a lower glycemic number, less processed, and higher in fiber.[3] And if you currently have any of the health risks we've mentioned, maintaining a diet of low to moderate glycemic foods will reduce your conditions and ultimately bring you back to a healthy functioning body. To motivate you to improve your food choices, remember that your body is in a constant state of breakdown and renewal. Ninety-eight percent of the atoms in your body will be completely replaced within one year.[4] Therefore the fuel you supply will change the atoms and structure from where you currently are, to where you want to be, and it starts right now.

The glycemic index is based on a sample of table sugar.[5] Table sugar is considered as having a high glycemic content as it is pure sugar and therefore it is given the number 100. By the way, white bread is also given the number 100[6] on the glycemic index which tells you a lot about how white bread affects your body – it is the same thing as eating pure sugar! All other foods are compared to this number and given their own number based on their sugar content. It breaks down as:

- Low GI foods (55 or less)
- Medium GI foods (56-69)
- High GI foods (70 and more)

One important note here: low glycemic foods don't necessarily mean they are healthy (Peanut M&Ms are a low glycemic food) and high glycemic foods don't necessarily mean they are unhealthy (watermelon is a high glycemic food). There are other factors that need to be considered when choosing a healthy food, and this includes:

- Fiber content
- Vitamins
- Minerals
- Calories

And finally, combining high glycemic healthy foods with low glycemic healthy foods (healthy protein and fat) will make the sugar take longer to hit your bloodstream and will assist with the glucose/insulin production and usage.

Carbohydrates are the primary energy source for the body. They are also the primary source of fuel for the brain.

There are four basic sugars which are called the simple carbohydrates:

- Glucose
- Lactose
- Fructose
- Sucrose

In order to eat right you need to consider the quality of the food you consume. The best choices are foods in their natural state, such as vegetables, fruits, proteins and whole grains. These foods are lower on the GI, they keep you satisfied longer and they provide nutrients your body requires to function properly. An important note here, don't confuse fructose with "high-fructose corn syrup." They are very different. Fructose is naturally occurring in foods such as fruit, where high-fructose corn syrup is a man-made sugar which is cheap to produce and has very harmful effects on the human body.

But in addition to learning where your food choice resides on the glycemic index scale, you also need to understand a term called glycemic load.

The Glycemic Load

Glycemic Load

Based on the glycemic index, the grams of available carbohydrate in the portion of food multiplied by the food's GI and divided by 100.

Glycemic load takes the *serving size* of your food into consideration.[7] If you locate the amount of carbohydrates in grams in a given food for the portion you are to consume, you would multiply that number by its glycemic value and then divide it by 100. This tells you how that serving of food will affect (or raise) your blood sugar by showing you *how much* you would have to consume to raise your blood sugar. Your blood sugar raises one gram of glucose for every one point of glycemic load. The glycemic load is measured in points.

If you eat a diet low in carbohydrates, you will automatically be eating foods with a low glycemic load.

A low glycemic load diet would be having less than 80 points for the day. A medium glycemic load is 80-120 points a day, and a high glycemic load would be over 120 points per day.[8]

This is important because a food that may seem high on the GI but have few carbohydrates per serving size could conceivably have a low glycemic load.

If a food has a glycemic load of 10 or less, it is considered low. If the glycemic load is 11 – 19, it's considered medium, and if it's 20 or more, it has a high load.

Some examples:

Watermelon has a GI of 76.[9] This is high on the glycemic index. But a cup of watermelon has only 11 grams of carbohydrates. So, 76 x 11= 836. Divide 836 by 100 and this food has a glycemic load of 8.36 which falls into a low glycemic load food.

White spaghetti has a GI of about 40.[10] This falls into the lower GI category. But it also has about 38 grams of carbohydrates per one cup serving. So, take the GI of 40 x

38 carbohydrates and that equals 1,520. Divide that by 100, and you get 15.2 putting it into the medium category of glycemic load.

How about good old french fries? French fries have a high glycemic index at 75[11] and the average serving of fries has about 38 grams of carbohydrate per serving. So, 75 x 38= 2850. Divide 2850 by 100 and that tells you that french fries have a very high glycemic index of 28.5. So, maybe next time you want to skip the fries and order a side of veggies or a salad. Now you know why our children and adults are becoming so obese with the "burger and fries" being an all American classic meal these days.

That's why you need to understand all of the components of your food.

Processed Food

There are two types of foods we can consume, whole foods and processed foods. Whole foods like fruits, vegetables, chicken, meat and fish are food in its natural state. Packaged, canned, and frozen foods are processed and mixed with substances to improve the flavor, preserve the food and often reduce the cost. These foods have labels and to know what you're eating and make your best choices, you need to learn to read labels.

The glycemic index or glycemic load is not on the label, but you can still find important facts on that label to help you make an educated choice. While you want to concentrate on foods that wind up with a low glycemic load, you also want to make sure you are getting nutritious foods as well. One popular nutritional program these days is called the "Paleo" diet stemming from the way that our paleolithic ancestors ate. One of the key factors of this nutritional program is that they did not consume "grains" in their diets because most grains are genetically modified and raise insulin and blood sugar levels in the body. We feel you should avoid grains in your diet as much as possible because of this, and the fact that it is very difficult to know which grains fall into this category since most grains come in packaged foods that are processed in a plant. Hence, this is why we believe that you should get your carbohydrates "from a plant" (fruits and vegetables) not from one *manufactured* "in a plant" (refined carbohydrates).

Food Labels

Calories in any food are made up of macronutrients called carbohydrates, proteins, fats, and sometimes alcohol (which is not a macronutrient). We utilize all of these elements for energy.

Calorie

The amount of energy a food contains.

We need to consume the appropriate number of healthy calories to maintain our ideal weight. One pound of fat is equal to about 3,500 calories. When we have consumed 3,500 more calories than we have expended, we will gain a pound of fat.[12] When we have used 3,500 calories more than the food we have consumed, our body will release the stored energy in our body, and we will lose a pound. In order to eat properly, and be able to use calories efficiently we have to know how many calories there are in the portion of food we're eating.

As mentioned, certain foods will satiate us better than others. When it comes to processed foods we need to look at the label to determine if that food is a good choice. A food may wind up sounding like a low calorie, low glycemic load food, but if the serving size is too small, you will not be satisfied long enough and that can lead to eating something else, maybe something that sabotages your best efforts.

Once you know the portion size and the calories per portion and feel that the portion size is adequate, you need to check a few other items.

The three most important things you'll need to know are:

- How much sugar is in the food
- The percentage and type of fat in the food
- How much fiber the food contains

When you look at a food label understand that the items are listed in order of quantity of that ingredient. The food contains the most of the first few ingredients and less of the items further down on the list. To put it in the simplest terms, if sugar is one of the first three ingredients, it has too much sugar. In addition to the listing of sugar, you may see high-fructose corn syrup, partially hydrogenated soybean oil or white flour as one of the first two ingredients. If so, don't buy it. We've already discussed that when food is excessive in sugar, the body cannot utilize it fast enough and therefore will store the extra sugar as fat.

An important word on HFCS (High Fructose Corn Syrup). HFCS is an "unnaturally" occurring, man-made sweetener.[13] It consists of a 55/45 ratio of fructose to glucose, where regular table sugar consists of a 50/50 ratio of fructose to glucose. Due to its chemical structure, HFCS does not need to be broken down or digested like regular table sugar and so our blood sugar spikes rapidly. Also, fructose triggers the liver into what is known as "lipogenesis," which is the production of fat by the liver. We believe that the switch from sugar to HFCS as a major sweetener in our food products has created much of the metabolic changes in our diets that have ultimately lead to the rapid rise in obesity, metabolic syndrome, diabetes, heart disease, and many other chronic conditions related to altered metabolism.

In recent history, we've gone from less than a pound (20 teaspoons) of sugar per person per year to about 150 pounds (4,800 teaspoons) of sugar per person per year. That's a half pound a day for every man, woman, and child in America. The average 20-ounce soda contains 15 teaspoons of sugar, all of it high-fructose corn syrup. And when you eat sugar in those doses, it becomes a toxin.[14]

Cane sugar and HFCS are NOT the same as we would be led to believe and HFCS should be avoided at all costs. Barry M. Popkin, Ph.D., Professor, Department of Nutrition, University of North Carolina at Chapel Hill has said "*The increase in consumption of HFCS has a temporal relation to the epidemic of obesity, and the over consumption of HFCS in calorically sweetened beverages may play a role in the epidemic of obesity.*"[15]

Fats in Processed Food

Fats are another important factor to understand. People often think that fat is bad for the body, but in truth, your body needs fats to survive. In fact, the Mediterranean cultures that consume a high fat diet but not a high carbohydrate diet are generally not only fitter than those of us who eat so many processed foods and refined carbohydrates, but they have fewer health issues.[16]

Fats are over twice as dense in calories than carbohydrates, proteins or alcohol and is the backbone behind many important structures in the body such as the brain, hormones and even the membranes of our cells.[17] So, when the fat consumed is a quality fat it satisfies you and you may wind up consuming fewer calories overall. But there are different types of fats in food. Therefore one rule of thumb is to try to limit your fat to no more than 30% of your total calories for the day. In addition, you need to stay away from the fats that are bad versus the fats that are good because fats like saturated fat and trans fats are known to be linked with serious life-threatening illness like cancer and heart disease.

One thing that you can do is read the labels on the food you're eating so you know what types of fats are in your food.

The good fats are:

- Monounsaturated/Omega 3 fatty acids
- Avocado
- Canola oil
- Cold water fish (like salmon)
- Flax seed oil
- Extra virgin coconut oil
- Soy products
- Nuts

These are the best forms of fats to ingest. They are not only healthy and necessary for the body, but include these potential benefits:

- Lower the risks of heart disease
- Reduce depression
- Prevent dementia
- Lower the risk of cancer
- Reduce arthritis
- Prevents inflammation
- Lower the risk for abnormal heart rhythm
- Slow plaque buildup inside blood vessels
- Lower triglycerides
- Lower high blood pressure
- Reduce the risk of stroke
- Reduction of allergies
- Reduction of eczema
- Improved memory[18,19]

Since the standard diet doesn't contain nearly high enough proportions of Omega 3 fats, supplements are highly beneficial. We recommend a high-quality, pharmaceutical grade fish oil if you are going to supplement. The supplement should be "distilled" for impurities since many impurities are stored in fat.

The next category is the fat that is less healthy, but not necessarily a bad fat. They are referred to as triglycerides because they contain three fatty acids and one glycerol. We call them neutral fats.

Neutral fats are:

- Saturated fats
- Fats from animal products
- Beef
- Cheese
- Butter

These fats are either solid at room temperature like butter and cheese or come from animal products. While we are categorizing these as neutral fats, they should only be used in moderation. Neutral fats serve as insulation. They conserve heat, protect the organs and are used for long term energy storage.

The worst fats are:

- Trans fat
- Solid margarine
- Hydrogenated oil

Trans fat are unnatural man-made fats and are used to improve the taste of food as well as preserve their shelf-life.[20] In the long run they are not worth the health risks.[21] Trans fat can raise bad cholesterol and lower good cholesterol. Both factors lead to the increased risks of metabolic syndrome.

You'll find the number of grams of trans fat on the nutrition label under the category 'fat'. If a product contains less than a half a gram of trans fat per serving, it may show a 0 in the trans fat gram count.[22] But be sure to check the ingredients list for any food made with hydrogenated oil or which says "partially hydrogenated" on the label because this means it does contain trans fat. So portion control is essential.

Trans fat is such a health risk that many of the fast food chains have stopped using hydrogenated oils in their production. Be wary though of any foods in restaurants where you cannot monitor the ingredients they use to prepare foods. Also, keep in mind that margarine is one of the worst offenders for containing trans fat.

Your brain is primarily made up of fat. When trans fat crosses the blood-brain barrier and takes residence in the brain, it alters transmission of nerve impulses leading to poor health and Alzheimer's disease.[23,24,25]

A recent article online at health.com includes the following list as some of the worst foods for trans fat as:

- French fries (particularly those fried in hydrogenated vegetable oils)
- Other fried or battered foods – (again particularly fried in hydrogenated vegetable oil)
- Pie and piecrust
- Sticks of margarine or similar other spreadable oil based sticks
- Shortening or lard
- Cake mixes and frostings
- Pancake and waffle mixes
- Fried chicken (fried in hydrogenated vegetable oil including frozen brands – so read the labels)
- Ice cream
- Non-dairy creamers
- Some microwaveable popcorns

We stress that you be vigilant and don't buy any product that lists partially or fully hydrogenated oil in the ingredient list.

7 Dietary Rules to Avoid Metabolic Syndrome

1. Plan your day. Each morning (or prior evening), sit down and plan your meals and record in a food diary or electronic app such as "my fitness pal". Planning and writing down your food choices is one of the most powerful things that you can do to change your eating habits.

2. Eat three meals and two snacks each day. Each meal should be no more than 300 calories unless your doctor recommends differently due to other circumstances such as a high amount of exercise training. Each of your three meals and two snacks per day should consist of a portion of carbohydrate, a portion of protein and a portion of fat. You can use a high-quality meal replacement shake for convenience for one or two of these meals or snacks.

3. Make healthy eating a priority. Enjoy your food and get back into the kitchen learning to cook healthy and use real food ingredients, avoiding processed, packaged and artificial food sources. Stop eating out so much, as the average meal eaten outside of the home is four times the amount of calories we need and loaded with ingredients that we have NO control over.

4. Be vigilant about serving sizes. Use this 'handy' guide to estimate the proper serving sizes: one serving of carbohydrate = 30 grams OR the size of your fist, one serving of protein = 20 grams OR the size of the palm of your hand and one serving of fat = 10 grams OR the size of your thumb.

5. Hydrate! Drink water every day. Do not dismiss this point. Water is the most abundant substance in your body, and you cannot function properly without it. Here's a tip: Consume half of your body weight in pounds in ounces of water; for example, if you weigh 150 lbs, consume at least 75 ounces of water per day. One trick is to bring a large glass of water with you to bed and leave it on your nightstand. Once you wake up, put your two feet on the floor, and greet your day with a replenishing glass of room temperature water. Drink another large glass with your two fish oil capsules and you are well on your way to consuming enough water for the day.

6. Caffeine is okay. Try to keep it to two cups per day. Stay away from all artificial sweeteners. If you need to sweeten your tea or coffee use regular sugar, but keep it to one teaspoon. You may also like the stevia sweeteners such as Truvia™ or Purvia™.

7. Don't drink your calories. Stay away from liquid calories such as juices, soda, diet soda or caloric drinks. Save your calories for real food. If you are trying to stick to the rule of no more than 300 calories per meal, it is very difficult to do if you are drinking your calories, and not leaving them for the food you want to consume.

When it comes to eating properly in this country, we've come to learn that "common sense isn't common practice." We believe one of the greatest things that you can do is to start to apply common sense to your eating habits. By bringing more awareness to your eating and drinking, you can radically change the way you look, the way you feel and ultimately the quality and quantity of your life. Start asking yourself (in a quiet voice to yourself), "should I eat this?", "is this going to give me energy or rob my energy?", "how am I going to feel two hours after I eat this?" When we take our eating habits from "unconscious" to "conscious" we can break the bonds of poor choice and addiction that have resulted in poor health. From this, we learn that power and vibrant health comes from making better and smarter nutritional decisions. In America, we've been given one of the greatest freedoms, the "freedom of choice." However, we must make sure that these same freedoms aren't making us unhealthy, obese and robbing us of the ability to live a long and healthy life. Freedom inherently comes with responsibility and one of the greatest responsibilities that we have is what we put into our mouths for this will ultimately shape our destiny and the destiny of those who love us.

8WW Success Story

"I feel better!
I look better!
I am better!"

Marge M.

When we began our first 8WW program together, my husband and I had no idea what to expect or how successful the program would be. What I did know is that I was certainly not as healthy as I could be and that my weight problem was close to overwhelming. At the end of the first 8WW program, we had been so successful that I knew I wanted and needed to do it again.

The weight on the scale now shows a 1/5 reduction from what it was when I started. I walk two miles at least three times a week. The weight training has dramatically increased my overall strength. The chiropractic adjustments keep me moving easily; the meditation classes and CDs help to keep me focused and relaxed; and the massage therapy is the best reward for hard work well done. I feel better; I look better; and, all the numbers in the blood work (lower cholesterol, lower blood sugar, etc.) show that I am better.

This was truly a team effort. The doctors and staff at the 8 Weeks to Wellness center are consistently enthusiastic, uplifting, and encouraging and personable. You all make the strenuous attainable and enjoyable through your heartfelt, confident approach to difficult goals.

Your slogan is right on the money – I gave you eight weeks, you changed my life!

8WW Success Story

Both Lost Over 25 Pounds!

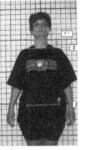

Regina Wallace
(with Dave Borsavage)

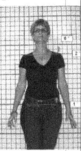

Dave and I started 8WW for improvement in his health. Dave is a diabetic and wanted to learn to eat better, lose weight, feel better and improve his lab numbers. I thought I was as healthy as I could be at 52 and going through menopause. I had tried a few weight loss programs in the last few years, and just watched my weight creep up. I had a few aches and pains (including extra weight) but thought I could not lose weight because of my hormones. I really wanted to support Dave in achieving his goals and inside I hoped I would lose just 10 pounds.

We followed the program, just like they said, "Just show up and it WILL work". That was in July. We planned menus on the weekend, shopped together and that made it easier to stay on track with the nutrition part. I have exercised in health clubs off and on throughout my years. How different could this be? I learned how to do exercises correctly with your guidance. You did challenge us to work out smarter, using heavier weights but always encouraging us.

We both have lost over 25 pounds each and feel great. Dave's A1c dropped one full point, he learned to work with you and even enjoyed the weekly massage. My little aches and pains have disappeared, the headaches and low back discomfort are gone and my posture has improved. My diet is better and my afternoon naps are not required. I actually feel 5 years younger. I have not been this thin since I met Dave 6 years ago.

Thank you 8 Weeks to Wellness, for giving us the "Back to Health" tools. It was a team lesson and "you are family".

Sources:

1. Jenkins, DJ et al. "Glycemic index of foods: a physiological basis for carbohydrate exchange." *The American journal of clinical nutrition* 34.3 (1981): 362-366.

2. "Glycemic index and glycemic load for 100+ foods - Harvard Health ..." 2005. 29 Dec. 2013 <http://www.health.harvard.edu/newsweek/Glycemic_index_and_glycemic_load_for_100_foods.htm>.

3. "What is the Glycemic Index? - The World's Healthiest Foods." 2003. 29 Dec. 2013 <http://www.whfoods.com/genpage.php?tname=faq&dbid=32>.

4. David Kestenbaum. "Atomic Tune-Up: How the Body Rejuvenates Itself : NPR." 2007. 29 Dec. 2013 <http://www.npr.org/templates/story/story.php?storyId=11893583>.

5. Ronald Roth. "Glycemic Index/Load + Simple-Refined-Complex Sugar/Carbs." 2002. 29 Dec. 2013 <http://www.acu-cell.com/gi.html>.

6. "GI Foods Advanced Search - Glycemic Index." 2011. 29 Dec. 2013 <http://www.glycemicindex.com/foodSearch.php.

7. "Glycemic index and glycemic load for 100+ foods - Harvard Health ..." 2005. 29 Dec. 2013 <http://www.health.harvard.edu/newsweek/Glycemic_index_and_glycemic_load_for_100_foods.htm>.

8. Laura Dolson. "What Is the Glycemic Load? - Low Carb Diets - About.com." 2005. 29 Dec. 2013 <http://lowcarbdiets.about.com/od/faq/f/faqgl.htm>.

9. Atkinson, Fiona S, Kaye Foster-Powell, and Jennie C Brand-Miller. "International tables of glycemic index and glycemic load values: 2008." *Diabetes Care* 31.12 (2008): 2281-2283.

10. Atkinson, Fiona S, Kaye Foster-Powell, and Jennie C Brand-Miller. "International tables of glycemic index and glycemic load values: 2008." *Diabetes Care* 31.12 (2008): 2281-2283.

11. Foster-Powell, Kaye, Susanna HA Holt, and Janette C Brand-Miller. "International table of glycemic index and glycemic load values: 2002." *The American journal of clinical nutrition* 76.1 (2002): 5-56.

12. "Counting calories: Get back to weight-loss basics - MayoClinic.com." 2005. 29 Dec. 2013 http://www.mayoclinic.com/health/calories/WT00011.

13. "Why You Should Never Eat High Fructose Corn Syrup Mark Hyman ..." 2013. 29 Dec. 2013 http://www.huffingtonpost.com/dr-mark-hyman/high-fructose-corn-syrup_b_4256220.html.

14. "Why You Should Never Eat High Fructose Corn Syrup Mark Hyman ..." 2013. 29 Dec. 2013 http://www.huffingtonpost.com/dr-mark-hyman/high-fructose-corn-syrup_b_4256220.html.

15. Bray, G.A., Nielsen, S.J., and B.M. Popkin. 2004. Consumption of high-fructose corn syrup in beverages may

play a role in the epidemic of obesity. *Am J Clin Nutr.* 79(4):537-43. Review.

16. "Mediterranean Diet -- What You Need to Know -- US News Best Diets." 2011. 29 Dec. 2013 <http://health.usnews.com/best-diet/mediterranean-diet>

17. "Energy density and weight loss: Feel full on fewer calories ..." 2005. 29 Dec. 2013 http://www.mayoclinic.com/health/weight-loss/NU00195.

18. "Omega-3 Slideshow: Benefits of Fish Oil, Salmon, Walnuts, & More." *WebMD.* Reviewed by: Brunlida Nazario, MD. WebMD, 21 Sept. 2012. Web.

19. "Major Trouble Ahead - If You Don't Fix This Deadly Deficiency." *Mercola.com.* N.p., 12 Jan. 2012. Web.

20. "Trans Fats - American Heart Association." 2010. 29 Dec. 2013 http://www.heart.org/HEARTORG/GettingHealthy/FatsAndOils/Fats101/Trans-Fats_UCM_301120_Article.jsp.

21. "Trans Fat Alert! 22 Foods to Watch - Health.com." 2011. 29 Dec. 2013 http://www.health.com/health/gallery/0,,20533295,00.html.

22. "What Are Trans Fats? Food Sources and Daily Limits - WebMD." 2008. 29 Dec. 2013 http://www.webmd.com/food-recipes/understanding-trans-fats.

23. "Brain Shrinkage? Trans Fats Link to Alzheimer's - Health & Science ..." 2012. 29 Dec. 2013 http://www.cbn.com/cbnnews/healthscience/2012/march/brain-shrinkage-trans-fats-link-to-alzheimers-/.

24. "Elderly Brains Stay Sharp After a Low Trans Fat Life |
LiveScience." 2011. 29 Dec. 2013
http://www.livescience.com/17664-brains-stay-sharp-trans-
fat.html.

25. Phivilay, A. "High dietary consumption of trans fatty
acids decreases brain ..." 2009.
<http://ww.ncbi.nlm.nih.gov/pubmed/19135506.

5

Mindful Based Stress Reduction

"To understand the immeasurable, the mind must be extraordinarily quiet, still." ~ Jiddu Krishnamurti

We've said so far that our goal is to teach you how to eat properly, move properly and think properly. So what do we mean when we say you need to *think* properly?

When we are faced with challenges, mishaps or life's irritations, the way we handle them has a direct impact on our health. Stress which is created, grown and fostered in the mind, causes depression and anxiety unless treated.[1] If we are in a happy, calm, relaxed state of mind, we will handle the stresses of life better. If we are happy and calm, we'll also be healthier. Stress in our body creates illness and disease. Researchers at Yale University have even shown that stress can cause sudden death.[2] Relaxation in your mind creates relaxation in your body and prevents stress and illness.[3] Look at the word 'disease'...*dis*-ease – when you are not at ease, you are not healthy.

In order to understand why prolonged stress is detrimental we need to look at the sympathetic nervous system, also called the *fight or flight response*. If we are in danger whether real or imagined, physical or psychological, our body goes into protection mode (to fight or flee). This will cause our pulse to race, our heart to beat faster, and our muscles to tighten and our immune system to shut down. This happens because the body now needs to focus all of its attention on dealing with the emergency situation. We have all experienced this feeling when we've had a near miss car accident or when we've taken a major test or given a public speech. Like the majority of our fears, the incident does not even have to be real. Have you ever had a bad dream, and then woken up to a racing heart, sweaty palms or quick breathing? This is your nervous system in fight or flight. Too many of us spend too many waking hours in some sort of panic.

Stress Related Conditions

If we remain in this heightened state of stress for extended periods or what we call "sustained sympathetic tone," our immune system is weakened and many of our bodily functions can become impaired. This can lead to a huge variety of health issues including: [4]

- Susceptibility to illness
- Digestive issues
- Sleep disturbances
- High blood pressure
- Depression
- Headaches
- Moodiness
- Poor concentration
- Memory problems
- Anxiety
- Constant worrying
- Feeling overwhelmed
- Negative thinking
- Eating disorders or problems
- Alcohol or drug addiction
- Nausea
- Rapid heartbeat
- Loss of libido
- Related aches and pains
- And more

Long-term stress, anxiety and depression have been linked with an increased risk of dementia and Alzheimer's disease. In fact, some research suggests that long-term stress stimulates the growth of the proteins that might cause Alzheimer's.That can lead to memory loss.

It also appears that the impact of stress on people's brain health is affected by other behaviors that can also harm the brain. Overeating, drinking alcohol and smoking cigarettes are among the informal stress management approaches people employ, but all of them increase the risk of damage to the brain in the form of a stroke.[5]

When we learn how to control our stress by applying a technique called mindful based stress reduction, or MBSR for short, we can change our external attitude and life experiences as well as our internal physiology and health conditions. MBSR is taught at many prestigious institutions such as the University of California[6], Duke University[7] and the University of Minnesota[8]. The great thing is that you do not have to go back to school to learn how to do this. It can be done at home, with just some time and energy on your part and some simple instruction.

People use mindful based stress reduction to help them deal with many issues including:[9]

- ADD/ADHD
- Anger/stress management
- Anxiety, panic, or depression
- Chronic pain
- Daily life stress
- Fatigue
- Headaches
- High blood pressure
- Job or family stress
- Personal growth and development
- Serious illness
- Sleep disturbances
- Type A behavior

In fact, one study revealed that people who were practicing mindful based stress reduction administered during light-treatment for psoriasis (an autoimmune skin disease) had four times the speed of healing for the chronic skin condition than those that had not practiced MBSR.[10]

Mindful based stress reduction is a technique where you quiet your mind and focus on your breath. You attempt to stop the chatter and thoughts that are constantly flooding your mind. You do this because when you focus on the current moment it is hard to worry about the past or the future. All you are thinking about is this moment, right now. We call this PTC, Present Time Consciousness. So you are not thinking about the payment that's due, or the work deadline, or the fight you had with your boss or the person that cut you off, or the financial crisis of the world...you leave all those stressors behind. When you are taught to focus on the present moment, you can often find peace and comfort. These feelings help you to feel more centered and happy. When you're more centered and happy, your body functions better.

The Effects of Reducing Stress

Think about it, when you feel love and joy you have a smile of your face and a bounce in your step. You don't sweat the small stuff. You do nice things for other people, just because it is the right thing to do! When you feel love and happiness you want to share it with others. So time spent feeling serene and peaceful is a way to lift your vibration to one that is closer to the feeling of love.

Mindful based stress reduction is a time you set aside for yourself. You sit quietly where you won't be disturbed and breathe slowly in and out. While slowly breathing like this you clear your mind from all thoughts. Your mind will naturally wander and thoughts will pop up. If you try to stop these thoughts you won't be able to relax, so just let them happen but don't concentrate on them. Instead, focus on the silence between the thoughts. When you 'stop thinking' you allow your mind and body to relax.

Sometimes guided audio programs are used to teach this technique of reducing your stress the healthy way. Doctors of Chiropractic that offer the 8WW program will provide this option. Mindful based stress reduction provides you with many benefits including improving brain function. These benefits as detailed in Meredith Melnicks research article published by the HuffingtonPost[11] include:

- Reducing stress and tension –emotionally and physically
- Reducing high blood pressure
- Reducing anxiety
- Reduction of depression
- Improving memory
- Improving concentration
- Improving critical thinking
- Elevating mood
- Reduced sensitivity to pain
- Increased happy feelings
- Less addictive tendencies
- Increased perspective and empathy
- Increased creativity
- Reduced concentration of C-reactive protein (associated with heart disease)

These benefits coincide with reduction in the conditions that lead to metabolic syndrome. In addition, mindful based stress reduction helps people make better, healthier choices about what they eat, whether they exercise and how they handle their relationships. Research even shows that MBSR is associated with improvements in mindful attention, emotion and well-being. These results continued for at least two months following the research and included improvements in moral reasoning and ethical decision making. This study provides preliminary evidence that MBSR may potentially facilitate moral reasoning and decision making in adults.[12]

Your attitude is important because it affects every aspect of your life. What you expect, you get. If you are having a 'bad day', you'll expect things to continue to go wrong. If you're in a bad mood, you're likely to snap at someone, and to make bad decisions and bad choices. If, on the other hand, you are feeling happy or having a good day, you will be able to overlook negative elements that may occur in the day, you'll handle challenges more easily, and you'll be more aware, more alert, and more patient.

In 2012 a study reported in *Frontiers in HUMAN NEUROSCIENCE* found that after an eight-week program of a variety of mindful-attention meditation training sessions, respondents showed enduring changes in health, psychological and brain functions. The study cites that these changes either cause or can lead to the following benefits[13]:

- A decrease in fearful responses to emotional stimuli
- Decreased depression
- Higher levels of compassion
- Significant reduction in self-criticism and shame
- Increase of positive, loving emotions
- Increased mindfulness
- Increased purpose of life
- Decrease of illness symptoms

- Increase in life satisfaction
- Improved emotion regulation

Can Stress Make You Fat?

What have you heard about stress, weight gain and cortisol?. Many of us have heard about this fat promoting hormone but don't really understand its effects or how it works against us. When you are under stress and haven't learned how to manage it in real time, powerful hormones such as adrenalin -- which gives us instant energy -- along with corticotrophin releasing hormone (CRH) and cortisol get released[14]. These hormones prepare our body to take action and release the appropriate energy and glucose to protect ourselves during flight or fight. However, most stressors these days do not require that we take immediate physical action such as run away, or climb up a tree as fast as possible, or lift a heavy object in order to clear a path to food or water. "Often, our response to stress today is to sit and stew in our frustration and anger, without expending any of the calories or food stores that we would if we were physically fighting our way out of stress or danger," says Shawn Talbott, PhD[15], an associate professor in the Department of Nutrition at the University of Utah and author of *The Cortisol Connection*.

Since our body doesn't know that we didn't work and expend energy it wants and needs to replenish the energy it thinks it just released, and so we get hungry after we go through the stress response. Hence, the relationship between stress and weight gain. The more disturbing problem is that when the body "re-stores" this energy, it does so as fat and it stores it around or mid-section or what is known as VAT- visceral adipose tissue.

Often this habit of being stressed and then reaching for our favorite fat or carbohydrate-ladened food is unconscious because we've been doing it for so long and don't even realize the connection anymore. But start paying attention to your habits when you are stressed and you may be surprised to realize that some of your most destructive health habits occur when you are stressed.

Stress Reduction and Metabolic Syndrome

The risk for weight gain and metabolic syndrome can be lessened when you raise your fitness level with exercise and reduce your stress levels with mindful based stress reduction techniques. But if you already have a serious illness, it is even more important to utilize this skill. Clinical trials have shown that mindful meditation has significant benefits to patients facing life-threatening illnesses. A study reported in Psychosomatic Medicine[16] showed that when they employed mindful based stress reduction, cancer patients with a wide variety of cancer diagnosis as well as varied stages of the disease had significantly lowered feelings of:

- Stress
- Depression
- Anxiety
- Anger
- Confusion

And

- Fewer cardiovascular issues
- Fewer gastrointestinal issues
- Less Irritability

- More energy
- Lowered symptoms of stress

More Stats

...mindfulness can do more than prevent a few gray hairs. According to (Kim) Dobson (MD), those who practice these techniques report dramatic improvements in health, a reduction in perceived chronic pain and improved immunity.

Participants also have displayed increased electrical activity and growth in areas of the brain that manage stress, tension and compassion.[17]

So with all these benefits, why aren't more people practicing MBSR? Some of it has to do with its relationship to meditation. Meditation is a sister to MBSR but tends to have religious components. MBSR is not and has nothing to do with your religious beliefs. It can and should be practiced by everyone, regardless of your faith. In our culture we are not taught MBSR in our schools or by our parents, yet. As the stresses of life increase and the complexities of the world increase we feel that it will be necessary to perform MBSR to be truly healthy. That is why it is included as a core part of our practice strategies.

8WW Success Story

Lost 26 Pounds!

Kim Buffington

What an honor to be chosen Patient of the Month. It means so much to me. And, it comes at a time in my wellness journey that I need to turn it up a notch. This honor gives me the boost that I need to continue forward. Thank you so much.

I thought about making this testimonial a cheeky little "Once upon a time, there was a little fat girl with a pretty face (if only she could get herself into shape to get that happily ever ending that every little girl wants)..." story. While that might be entertaining, it also might be disrespectful to those that have played such an amazing part in my journey. So instead, I'll just be truthful because being truthful is what it takes to heal yourself no matter what your obstacle is. Step one for me, recognizing the problem.

A little over a year ago, my mirror suddenly became truthful, or maybe it was my eyes, and I saw for the first time what others were seeing when looking at me. I was horrified, not just for the way I looked but for the health issues that were starting to present themselves to me. Being overweight was not a surprise because I have battled the scale my entire life. What was horrifying was how out of control I had become despite a lifetime of "good efforts". I thought seriously about what my future could possibly hold if I continued with the same old same old. It certainly could never be happy or productive. I considered all of the failed efforts and wondered what went wrong. I finally recognized that I didn't have the tools or knowledge to fix this myself otherwise how could this have happened in the first place? So, what's the plan then?

Look over there...it's Jim O'Malley! How lucky for me to have him as a colleague and friend. Jim you are an inspiration beyond belief and always so supportive; I am forever grateful to you. I watched Jim change his life and now I'm working to change mine.

(continued on next page)

8WTW Success Story

Lost 26 Pounds!

Kim Buffington

(continued from previous page)

Jim introduced me to 8 Weeks to Wellness where I was brought to tears with your insight and honesty. You made me realize that I needed to make myself the priority in my life otherwise, who else would? My job to do, check. This job is a big one. One that requires a lot of hard work and dedication.

How can I have the dedication needed to take on this huge task? Easy, surround yourself with caring, supportive allies. Thanks for keeping me aligned. For your helpful suggestions and for easing my pain. I was terrified at first but now can't wait to see you. You should know by now that I brag on two continents about you. Also for helping me see the big picture and to appreciate all of the little things that make up the big picture.

Thank you to the entire team, for your support, advice, and magic hands...thank you for healing me. Thanks for keeping an eye on me and stepping in when needed. You all are inspirational and motivating and I am happy to see your faces every time I step into the gym.

You make it possible for me to step forward each day and try to make myself a better person. Thank you for your patience, your knowledge, your effort and for never giving up on me.

Thank you for being hard & strong when I needed it, and being silly when I need it even more. Thank you for expecting more from me than I would ever dare to expect of myself. You rock!

Thank you for saving my life.

8WW Success Story

Lost 47 Pounds!
Body Fat
Before: 44.1% *After:* 37.2%
BP Diastolic
from 90 to 70
Glucose
From 125 to 95
Triglycerides/HDL Ratio
from 6.36 to 2.37
Health Satisfaction:
Before: 65 points,
After: 140 points

Gail

While I was recovering from surgery, not able to do much, I was reading the newspaper and came across an ad that read "8 Weeks to Wellness!" It went on to describe losing weight, dropping your blood sugar and losing inches all without medication - yeah right!! But then the program goes on to say they include a full health assessment with chiropractic adjustments and massages among other things. So I thought what the heck, I've tried how many diets and workout programs and I still need to change so I made the call. I am so thankful that I did!!

From my first contact to schedule my orientation which I rescheduled a couple of times, to me finally meeting with the Wellness family I was hooked. They gave me the confidence to begin my journey.

So on we went with my initial assessment and my team came up with my game plan. Before you knew it we were at 8 weeks and 25 pounds lighter, all my counts were down and I was able to do stretches and exercises that I haven't done in years. Their encouragement and friendship kept me going.

(continued on next page)

8WW Success Story

Lost 47 Pounds!

Body Fat
Before: 44.1% *After:* 37.2%
BP Diastolic
from 90 to 70
Glucose
From 125 to 95
Triglycerides/HDL Ratio
from 6.36 to 2.37
Health Satisfaction:
Before: 65 points,
After: 140 points

Gail

(continued from previous page)

I am currently in my 18th week, 47.2 pounds lighter and I feel like a new person. After years of numerous diets and going to workout centers this new family helped heal my whole body and spirit through bi-weekly workouts, chiropractic adjustments, massages, teaching me new eating habits and meditation.

Since the first day, the constant support, encouragement, motivation and friendship has helped carry me through.

I just wanted to let you all know how important and special you have made me feel.

Thank you from the bottom of my heart. You are not done with me yet - see you next week.

Sources:

1. David DiSalvo. "Stress Kills The Mind, One Day At A Time - Forbes." 2013. 22 Dec. 2013
http://www.forbes.com/sites/daviddisalvo/2013/05/30/stres
s-kills-the-mind-one-day-at-a-time/.

2. "Yet Another Reason to Avoid Stress: Sudden Death - WebMD." 2010. 22 Dec. 2013
http://www.webmd.com/balance/stress-
management/news/20000117/yet-another-reason-avoid-
stress-sudden-death.

3. Carlson, Linda E et al. "One year pre–post intervention follow-up of psychological, immune, endocrine and blood pressure outcomes of mindfulness-based stress reduction (MBSR) in breast and prostate cancer outpatients." Brain, behavior, and immunity 21.8 (2007): 1038-1049.

4. "Stress Symptoms, Signs & Causes: Effects of Stress Overload." 2003. 22 Dec. 2013
http://www.helpguide.org/mental/stress_signs.htm.

5. "Discovery Health "Effect of Stress on the Brain"." 2010. 22 Dec. 2013
http://health.howstuffworks.com/wellness/stress-
management/effect-of-stress-on-the-brain.htm.

6. "Mindfulness Based Stress Reduction (MBSR) at UC San Diego ..." 2012. 22 Dec. 2013
http://health.ucsd.edu/specialties/mindfulness/mbsr.

7. "Mindfulness-Based Stress Reduction - Duke Integrative Medicine." 2011. 22 Dec. 2013 http://www.dukeintegrativemedicine.org/classes-workshops-and-education/mindfulness-based-stress-reduction.

8. "Mindfulness-Based Stress Reduction - Center for Spirituality and ..." 2013. 22 Dec. 2013 http://www.csh.umn.edu/workshops-and-lectures/mindfulness-based-stress-reduction/index.htm.

9. "Current Research Studies - Duke Integrative Medicine." 2011. 22 Dec. 2013 http://www.dukeintegrativemedicine.org/research/current-research-studies.

10. "MBSR and psoriasis | Wildmind Buddhist Meditation." 2007. 22 Dec. 2013 http://www.wildmind.org/applied/stress/mbsr/mbsr-abstract02.

11. Melnick, Meredith. "Meditation Health Benefits: What The Practice Does To Your Body." The Huffington Post. TheHuffingtonPost.com, 30 Apr. 2013.

12. Shapiro, SL. "Mindfulness-based stress reduction effects on moral reasoning." 2012. http://www.tandfonline.com/doi/abs/10.1080/17439760.2012.723732.

13. Desbordes, Gaelle, Lobsang T. Negi, Thaddeus W. W. Pace, B. Alan Wallace, Charles L. Raison, and Eric L. Schwartz. "Effects of Mindful-attention and Compassion Meditation Training on Amygdala Response to Emotional Stimuli in an Ordinary, Non-meditative State." Frontiers. Frontiers in Neuroscience, 2012.

14. Can Stress Cause Weight Gain? May 13th, 2005 WebMD-http://www.webmd.com/diet/features/can-stress-cause-weight-gain.

15. Talbott; "The Cortisol Connection" 2007. Hunter House Publishers.

16. Speca, Michael, PsyD, Linda E. Carlson, PhD, Eileen Godney, MSW, and Maureen Angen, PhD. "A Randomized, Wait-List Controlled Clinical Trial: The Effect of a Mindfulness Meditation-Based Stress Reduction Program on Mood and Symptoms of Stress in Cancer Outpatients." Pyschosomatic Medicine Journal of Behavioral Medicine, 2013.

17. Robinson, Marcene. "UB Faculty and Staff Are Welcome to Relax in Mindfulness Meditation Course." - News Center. University at Buffalo The State University of New York, 4 Sept. 2013. Web.

6

Massage

"The physician must be experienced in many things, but most assuredly in rubbing." -**Hippocrates**, The "Father of Modern Medicine"

Massage Is Necessary

When most people hear that massage is one of the vital elements of the 8 Weeks to Wellness® program they get excited (or confused). Massage is quite often believed to be simply a pampering luxury. A gentle massage at a spa may be exactly that, but the massage we require has some additional necessary functions.

Because our program requires you to repeatedly exercise to your maximum efficiency, your body is intentionally working much harder than it is used to. When you exercise the correct way you increase your circulation, bringing more oxygen and energy to your muscles so that they can perform. The byproduct of this performance is toxins, such as lactic acid, and other spent fuel that can build up in your muscles.[1,2] Eventually the toxins leave your muscles and move on to your liver, kidney, spleen and lungs where they will be excreted from your body. Without the *deep tissue toxin releasing* massage, you will be leaving those toxins in your muscles too long. If they are not removed they can have serious effects.

Some signs of accumulating toxins and lowered health include:

- Discharge from the eyes, nose or ears.
- Appearance of pigmentation or inflammatory lesions such as skin rashes, pustules, acne, or gum disease.
- Loss of energy, weakness or physical trouble with exercise. When we exercise some discomfort can be felt as minor damage occurs and is repaired for future exercise. This is conditioning and is normal. When you begin exercising gently and gradually increase the intensity of effort, you will feel improvement. Exercise can also release toxins that

are stored in fatty and other connective tissues. Once released these toxic compounds can cause signs and symptoms of disease as they negatively affect their target tissues. Exercise or movement that is too aggressive in toxic people can lead to serious issues. Toxic-laden patients often dislike exercise as their body is instructing them not to move so they will keep these toxins hidden in their tissues. Such people should discuss their condition with their medical professionals.

- Weight gain. Eating a calorie-restricted diet improves many health factors and may even extend life. Obesity aggravates many health issues. Did you know that fat is the body's reaction to a toxic situation? Excessive glucose made from ingesting too many calories would be damaging to the body, and while we need sugar for our cells to operate properly, excessive amounts are harmful. The body will store fat-soluble toxins like pesticides in fatty deposits. When we exercise those toxins can be released and make us feel poorly. It is interesting how many people and pets lose weight easily once their undergo detoxification therapy.

- Aches and pains or muscle wasting can signal the accumulation of toxins. When we exercise the tissues release toxic materials and if these accumulate then we feel poorly. Conditioning and eating properly helps improve the health of our lymphatic and blood vessels and this makes us more efficient at removing toxins.

- Poor digestion. Toxins negatively affect the normal structures of our digestive organs, and this can lead to stomach and bowel upsets, diarrhea, gas and constipation. If digestion is incomplete then residual materials accumulate and provide food and shelter for undesirable bacteria, fungi and yeasts. These

can trigger inflammatory reactions locally and globally. This can be minimized by including fresh non-starchy vegetables in the diet.[3]
- Difficulty sleeping can be related to toxin accumulation and organ dysfunction.[4]

Massage moves the toxins from your muscles and gets them into the blood system where they can be transported and broken down by the organs and released. Massage therefore is necessary.

Many hospitals and even children's hospitals[5], institutions and even mental health hospitals[6] are incorporating massage into their programs because of the many benefits. Gone are the days of massage being considered an unnecessary luxury for the ultra elite.Therapeutic massage is vital for true health. While reading this book, take your hand that is not holding the book and reach up to your opposite shoulder. With two fingers push down into the space between your shoulder and your neck closer to your neck. You won't have to push very hard to feel the accumulation of stress that causes you pain. Even with light pressure this area is very sensitive to most. The problem is you are so used to it, you didn't even know it is there! Once you have a therapeutic massage and that stress is relieved you will discover how that stress was affecting your feelings, behaviors, choices and your relationships.

As far as our requirements, the massage should be performed by a licensed massage therapist. They will have the ability to report back to your doctors and trainer to let us know how sore and tight you are and the amount of toxins you have. This lets us know how hard you are working, and allows us to adjust the program.

In a moment we'll explain a little more about massage, but we do want you to follow these simple steps in conjunction with our recommendations:

- Schedule a one hour massage each week.
- Bath or shower prior to the massage preferably as close to the massage time as possible. This removes all toxins from your skin and begins to relax the muscles, tendons and ligaments.
- Do not exercise the same day.
- Drink plenty of water after the massage to assist the body in eliminating the toxins from the blood and organs.

Benefits of Massage

Everyone knows that a massage will relax you and allow you to move more comfortably because any tightness you had will be decreased. But the type of massage we prescribe has more important benefits, including:

- Moving toxins out of the muscles
- Increasing circulation
- Aiding recovery from strenuous activity
- Enhancement of athletic performance
- Reduction of muscular tension
- Monitoring level of activity and efficiency
- Reducing hypertension
- Stress reduction
- And more

What Is Massage?

There are a great many different massage techniques and each is used for a different purpose. In general, massage is the hands-on manipulation of the tissues and muscles in the body in order to create a variety of health benefits.[7] Since you are forcing your body to work hard during your exercise sessions you will often be sore afterwards, but don't worry, it's a good kind of soreness. When you feel sore from your workout, it's a badge of honor you have earned because you know your body is getting stronger, healthier, more fit and functioning at its best. However, in order to continue to get the most out of your exercise regime as well as to benefit you as much as possible, you need to assist your body, muscles and tissues in recovering so they can get stronger. The massage helps you to achieve this.

The massage we most often prescribe is often known as a deep tissue massage because the licensed therapist is working deep into the tissues to release the toxins, relax the muscles and improve your range of motion. This prevents your muscles from getting too tight and your joints from becoming too stiff, both of which would make your next workouts less effective. It will also allow your body to recover from the work you've just done more quickly and will help to lessen the soreness you'll encounter.[8] This type of therapeutic massage also helps to stimulate endorphins[9], the same opiod peptides that a great workout will produce. This not only can make you feel happier, more energetic, and produce a sense of well-being, it's also a natural painkiller. Endorphins are natural hormones that are stored in the pituitary gland and are released by exercise as well as deep tissue stimulation as in a massage.[10] This is one of the reasons why a great workout regardless of the resulting soreness feels so rewarding.

The Difference Is Important

There is a real and important difference between getting a massage from a licensed massage therapist and a non-licensed (certified) massage therapist. A certified massage therapist has a certificate which attests that the individual has demonstrated a certain level of mastery of a specific body of knowledge and skills within the relevant field of practice. Certification should not be confused with either licensing or accreditation. While each involves some type of evaluation and the awarding of some type of credential, they are quite different from one another and the terms should not be used interchangeably.[11]

Licensing grants permission to an *individual* to engage in an occupation if it finds that the applicant has attained the degree of competency required to ensure the public health, safety, and welfare will be reasonably protected.

Certification differs from licensing in that it is nearly always offered by a private, non-governmental agency. Such agencies are usually outgrowths of professional associations which create certifying agencies to identify and acknowledge those who have met a standard.

Another contrast with licensure is that, under a licensing law, practitioners of the licensed occupation must have a license in order to practice. It is involuntary. On the other hand, certification is voluntary. One does not have to be certified in order to practice. An individual takes the certification exam because they want to enjoy the benefits of certification. However, to use the title and initials copyrighted and associated with the professional certification, one must be certified.[12]

Each state varies, but in general a non-licensed therapist will perform a relaxation massage versus a therapeutic massage. A relaxation massage is commonly what you get on vacation or on a cruise ship. While these can feel great, they are not the same as a therapeutic massage. The relaxation massage is soft and soothing massage and will relax you, has no real long-lasting medical benefit. This type of massage can be given by a loved one or from a masseuse with little formal technical training.[13]

A licensed massage therapist, on the other hand, will perform a therapeutic massage. This type of massage has a defined goal for the client and is administered by a trained professional. The goals of a therapeutic massage are to:[14,15,16]

- Release toxins from muscle groups
- Mobilize tight joints
- Relax tight muscles
- Relax muscles around the joints
- Restore range of motion
- Create greater flexibility of joints
- Remove toxins from lymphatic areas

Licensed Massage Therapists

A masseuse who is licensed has an advanced clinical and technological understanding of the body. These therapists will have a minimum of 500 hours and can have as much as 1,000 hours of supervised in-class initial massage therapy training. This training will include the study of many of the following:[17]

- Anatomy
- Physiology
- Pathology
- Nutrition

- Kinesiology
- Ethics
- Structure and function of the body
- Theory and practice of massage therapy
- Assessment and treatment techniques
- Hydrotherapy
- Homeopathy
- Breathing and stretching techniques
- CPR and first aid
- And most likely some elective subjects

Licensed massage therapists have learned about the structure of the human body. They know the names of the bones and muscles as well as their functions. They understand how the bones and muscles interact and they understand the different conditions that would require a specific technique for a problem, or for additional benefits to their client.

The massage may be a bit uncomfortable at times while the therapist works on your muscles but this is necessary in order to provide the eventual relief as well as accelerate the removal of the cells' waste. When your muscles are tight, it is more difficult for the toxins to get out and move through the blood system. When you exercise, you have increased the amount of toxin that needs to be released. A massage will open up the muscles, creating larger areas for the toxins to move out of the muscles, tissues, etc. and flow into the bloodstream in order to allow the body to excrete them. It helps when you drink water to hydrate your body providing more fluid to move the toxins out of your body.

What Can a Licensed Massage Therapist Ascertain During Your Massage?

We've mentioned that your massage therapist will report back to your trainer and doctors. You may wonder what they might be telling us and how they know what they know. Since a licensed therapist has extensive training in physiology, they can determine what is going on with your body from the act of the massage. A report to us might say something like this:

"Donna has got a lot of tightness and spasms in her latissimus dorsi muscle or pectoral muscles that she wasn't even aware of until I started massaging the area. I was amazed at the number of trigger points and the heightened sensitivity she had there, what's going on with her in the training center?"

And the trainer may report back that they just began a new exercise like the TRX straps that uses muscles that haven't been worked in that manner previously. In this type of communication you will be monitored to ensure that any pain or spasm or tightness will taper off as your muscles adapt to the new exercise. It all works together in unison.

Toxins and Massage

When we use the term toxins we are talking about the soreness you feel after a workout. Ever have the delayed reaction, a day or two after your workout, where your legs hurt, especially when walking down stairs? Or when you lift your arm to brush your hair, and that movement is suddenly difficult? This is because when you exercise a muscle, you are breaking down that muscle.[18] This leads to acid buildup[19] which is lessened when you cool down properly after a workout. If you don't cool down properly or your cool down is too quick or abrupt, the acid turns into acidic crystals. This is what you're feeling when you are sore a day or so later. The muscle fibers are moving against the acidic crystals and are slightly breaking as they move back and forth. A proper cool down will minimize the crystal formation, but even so there will still be some crystals that need to be moved out of your system by a therapeutic massage.

The level of toxins you have can often be quantified by the amount of soreness you feel, or how restrictive your muscles are. The therapist can determine that you have excess toxins by the severity of the spasms or number of trigger points they find. The more toxins you have, the more severe the level of soreness you'll have in a given area. This will also happen as you change your workout routine. When you use muscles in a new manner, you will feel the residual effects.

Having a therapeutic massage and the feedback from your licensed massage therapist allows you to progress properly, quickly and safely. Massage is a necessary and huge part of the Chiropractic lifestyle.

8WW Success Story

Lost 26 Pounds!

Debby Cipolloni

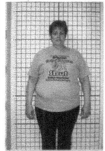

I had tried losing weight for quite some time.
Everything I tried just wasn't working. Then I was
introduced to The 8 Weeks to Wellness program. Little did
I know how much my life was about to change.

I knew I wasn't in the best of health when I came in for my
initial exam. But after my "Report of Findings" appointment,
I found out exactly how unhealthy I really was. As the doctor
went over my report of findings and my wellness score, I
was actually fighting back tears. I was determined before,
but now sitting in the office, I became absolutely committed
to changing my life and how I was living it.

I began the 8 Weeks to Wellness program on May 13th,
2013. The program taught me how to eat the right foods
in the proper amounts. The orientation and "How to Eat
Right for Life" workshop were also extremely helpful. You
explained how Chiropractic played such an important role
in optimum health and always had words of encouragement
for me when I came in for my bi-weekly adjustments. Your
staff always had words of encouragement as well.

When it came to the training portion of the program, I was
nervous. I hadn't worked out in about a year and a half and
had put on a lot of weight. I didn't know what I was going to
be able to do. The staff made me feel comfortable the first
time I walked in the gym. You started me out with what you
knew I would be able to do even if I had to just push myself
to do it.

(continued on next page)

8WW Success Story

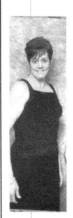

Lost 26 Pounds!

Debby Cipolloni

(continued from previous page)

Throughout the 8 weeks, you were supportive but pushed me as far as I needed to be pushed. And that is what helped me to be as successful as I was on the program.

And the massage, well all I have to say about that portion is AWESOME! Who doesn't enjoy a good massage? And your team certainly made mine enjoyable and relaxing. Their hands can do magic!!

At the end of the 8 weeks, I had lost 26 pounds. But along with the weight loss, I felt better than I had felt in years. I had dropped my dosage of Nexium from twice a day down to once a day and one of the other medications I was on I began weaning off.

I don't know how to thank everyone at 8WW for helping me and supporting me as I continue my journey along the road to optimum health. You all have made me feel like I'm part of one big family from day 1 and I greatly appreciate it!

8WEW Success Story

"I lost 17 pounds and 4 inches off my waist!"

Eddie Guster

AWESOME!! If I could stand on top of a mountain and shout out about 8 Weeks to Wellness®, I would. After feeling fat and sick of being out of breath every time I wanted to play sports, I looked at my wife and said, "it is time to make a change". My wife agreed and we found your 8 Week to Wellness® program.

After starting to lose weight, everyone was asking me what diet program I was on. I told them I am on no diet program, but a lifestyle changing program. Eight Weeks to Wellness has taught me how to change my lifestyle so that I can enjoy a healthy, happy life.

I lost 17 pounds and four inches off my waist. I fit in clothes that haven't fit for years. I FEEL GREAT!!! I can't thank you and the staff of 8 Weeks to Wellness® enough for all that you have done for me. I recommend this program for anyone who is serious about changing their lifestyle, losing weight and feeling good. It has changed my life and I look forward to continuing what I learned during my 8 week program.

Thanks for Everything!

Sources:

1. "Dr. Richard Palmquist: Toxins and Exercise - Huffington Post." 2012. 22 Dec. 2013 http://www.huffingtonpost.com/richard-palmquist-dvm/signs-of-systemic-toxin-a_b_1214624.html.

2. "Why Do Muscles Ache After Exercise? - Blurtit." 2013. 22 Dec. 2013 http://health.blrtit.com/104025/why-do-muscles-ache-after-exercise.

3. http://www.kotsanisinstitute.com/services/digestive-disorders.

4. "Dr. Richard Palmquist: Toxins and Exercise - Huffington Post." 2012. 22 Dec. 2013. <http://www.huffingtonpost.com/richard-palmquist-dvm/signs-of-systemic-toxin-a_b_1214624.html.

5. "Massage Therapy : Nationwide Children's Hospital." 2010. 22 Dec. 2013 http://www.nationwidechildrens.org/massage-therapy.

6. "new research supports the mental health benefits of massage therapy." 2013. 22 Dec. 2013 http://www.multivu.com/mnr/63936-amta-massage-therapy-research-roundup-mental-health-benefits.

7. "Massage - Definition and More from the Free Merriam-Webster ..." 2006. 22 Dec. 2013 http://www.merriam-webster.com/dictionary/massage.

8. "Massage: Get in touch with its many benefits - MayoClinic.com." 2005. 22 Dec. 2013 http://www.mayoclinic.com/health/massage/SA00082.

9. Kaada, Birger. "Increase of plasma β-endorphins in connective tissue massage." *General Pharmacology: The Vascular System* 20.4 (1989): 487-489.

10. "Exercise and Depression: Endorphins, Reducing Stress, and More." 2007. 22 Dec. 2013 http://www.webmd.com/depression/guide/exercise-depression.

11. "Credentials for the Massage Therapy Profession — American ..." 2004. 22 Dec. 2013 http://www.amtamassage.org/findamassage/credential.html.

12. "Credentials for the Massage Therapy Profession — American ..." 2004. 22 Dec. 2013 http://www.amtamassage.org/findamassage/credential.html.

13. "Credentials for the Massage Therapy Profession — American ..." 2004. 22 Dec. 2013 http://www.amtamassage.org/findamassage/credential.html.

14. Smith, MC et al. "Benefits of massage therapy for hospitalized patients: a descriptive and qualitative evaluation." *Alternative therapies in health and medicine* 5.4 (1999): 64.

15. "Massage Benefits: 9 Healthy Reasons To Make An Appointment ..." 2012. 22 Dec. 2013 http://www.huffingtonpost.com/2012/02/08/massage-benefits-health_n_1261178.html.

16. "The benefits of massage therapy." 2013. 22 Dec. 2013 http://www.usatoday.com/story/life/weekend/health/doctors/2013/12/20/benefits-of-massage-therapy/4137819/.

17. "Credentials for the Massage Therapy Profession —
American ..." 2004. 22 Dec. 2013
http://www.amtamassage.org/findamassage/credential.html.

18. Yarasheski, KEVIN E, JEFFREY J Zachwieja, and
DENNIS M Bier. "Acute effects of resistance exercise on
muscle protein synthesis rate in young and elderly men
and women." American Journal of Physiology-
Endocrinology And Metabolism 265.2 (1993): E210-E214.

19. Maltais, Francois et al. "Oxidative capacity of the
skeletal muscle and lactic acid kinetics during exercise in
normal subjects and in patients with COPD." American
journal of respiratory and critical care medicine 153.1
(1996): 288-293.